By reading this document, the reader agrees that under no circumstances is the author responsible for any losses, direct or indirect, which are incurred as a result of the use of information contained within this document, including, but not limited to, — errors, omissions, or inaccuracies.

Contents

Introduction

Congratulations!

You have taken the first step toward living a healthy lifestyle! If you are here today, you've probably been having trouble losing weight. We've all been there, and felt the frustration.

I tried Weight Watchers, Jenny Craig, and every calorie-counting, low-fat diet you can think of.

It never seemed to work, and I was always tired, hungry and miserable. Not only did the diets not work, it seemed like I kept *gaining* weight, the more time that went on and the more I tried to follow low fat diets.

Does any of this sound familiar?

If it does, you're not alone. We've been misled about diet and nutrition for decades. The medical establishment got tricked into believing that a low-fat diet was the key to health, and all we needed to do was count calories and limit portion sizes.

It turns out that all of the advice the experts have been giving us for decades is completely wrong. Discovered nearly by accident, the ketogenic diet does the exact opposite of what the nutrition experts have been saying. It's a high-fat diet that doesn't limit portion sizes or leave you feeling hungry. Rather than counting calories, this diet is based on limiting carbohydrates like sugar and starches. It turns out that it's carbs that cause weight gain. If you want to lose fat, you eat fat!

Since most people have been eating a high-carb diet laden with sugar for their entire lives, the keto diet can be quite a change. Shifting your eating habits like that without a guide to show you the right way to do it can be difficult and intimidating.

And that's why I've written this book. In this book I am going to explain in plain English what the keto diet is and how it's going to benefit your health, while helping you to lose weight rapidly. Then I am going to go into the details, telling you exactly what you can eat and what to avoid. We'll also discuss how to overcome common problems that come with starting the keto diet, as your body adjusts to this new way of eating. We'll give beginner tips, and talk about keto and diabetes. Then we'll discuss intermittent fasting – which is taking the world by storm as a way to improve health and help with weight loss. It turns out that intermittent fasting works just like the keto diet, and they are complimentary to each other. Finally, I'm going to give you a 21-day meal plan with a few recipes to help you get started.

Put simply, this diet works, and it keeps the weight off!

Chapter 1: What is Keto?

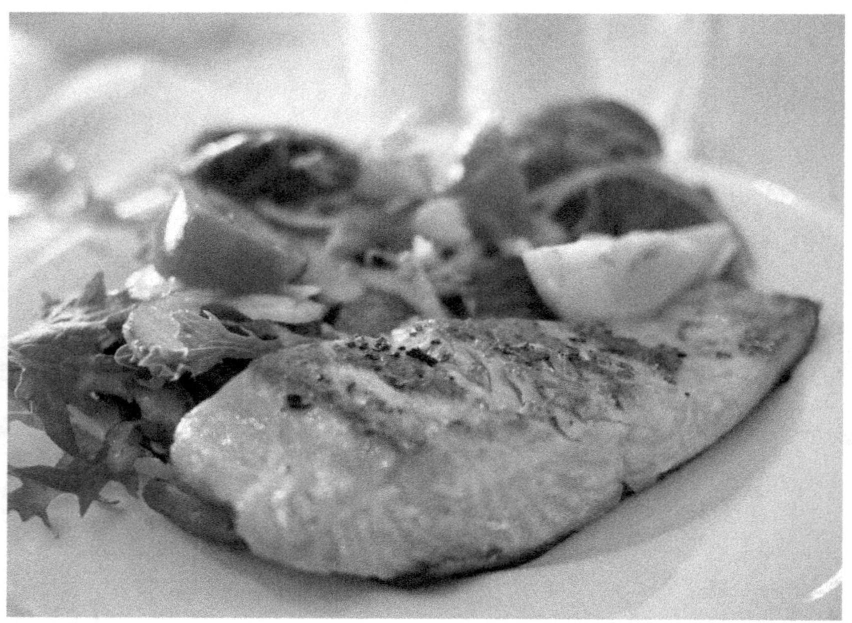

You've heard all the hype, but what is the keto diet and where did it come from? In this chapter we're going to give you a quick history of the keto diet, and how it came to be. It turns out that the keto diet was not developed for weight loss, but that turned out to be one of its biggest benefits that was discovered by accident. After we find out where the keto diet came from, we'll briefly discuss how it works, and go into more detail about this in the next chapter.

The History of the Keto Diet

Later we'll see that the ketogenic diet has a lot in common with fasting, on a physiological basis. So, it's not really accidental that the ketogenic diet originally gained favor as a treatment for epilepsy. If you go back in history, you'll find that the ancients recognized that fasting could help to mitigate the symptoms of epilepsy, but they didn't understand how it worked. Nonetheless, Hippocrates and others described the benefits of fasting for treating and managing epilepsy.

This ancient knowledge was largely forgotten for centuries. Fast forward to the early 20th century, and medical researchers began reinvestigating the role of fasting in the treatment of epilepsy. In 1911, research conducted in France revealed that epilepsy patients that ate a low-calorie diet that incorporated periodic fasting had fewer epileptic seizures, and they were able to manage them better.

This information caught on in the United States, and early efforts at using diet to treat epilepsy focused on using several days of fasting. There is no question that it helped epileptic patients reduce fasting, however people began to wonder if there was a better way to get the same benefits. This movement was also spurred by the fact that when epileptic patients went off the fasting, the previous level of seizures returned. So, it was clear that there was something beneficial about fasting, but it didn't have a permanent effect. As a result, medical researchers began to wonder what it was about fasting that was making the difference. Was its simple deprivation of calories, or something else? And if they could find the answer, is there some way that fasting could be mimicked, or was there another way to put the body into the fasting state?

Research conducted at the Mayo clinic found the answer. They discovered that epileptic seizures were reduced when blood sugar levels were lower due to restricted consumption of carbohydrates. At the time, physicians didn't completely understand all the hormones in the body and how they worked with digestion and the fasting state, but they were able to make the connection between blood sugar levels and epileptic seizures. In order to enable patients to avoid having to fast all the time, a physician Dr. Peterman developed a diet that limited carbohydrates while emphasizing a high fat diet, so that patients would be able to maintain lower blood sugars. The goal was to mimic the metabolic state the body goes into while fasting. Dr. Peterman believed that this diet would keep the body in a perpetual fasted state, and therefore help to control epilepsy without requiring patients to fast.

Peterman developed a diet that used a ratio of 4:1 of fat to protein and carbs. This type of diet is a little extreme compared to the modern version of the keto diet, getting 90% of the calories from fat. As we'll see later, while you will be eating a lot fatter than you're used to, it's not nearly the level that was originally prescribed for the diet used to control epilepsy.

Unfortunately, the use of this diet to treat epilepsy remained obscure and never caught on with the general public, largely because anti-convulsant drugs were developed that led doctors to use medications rather than diet to treat epilepsy. In the interim, after World War II the American medical establishment and government began pushing a high-carbohydrate and low-fat diet. In part, this push came about as a result of the research by one man, Dr. Ancel Keyes. He did a study that is commonly referred to as the seven countries study, which claimed to study the diet eaten in each of the seven countries looking for clues to the cause of heart disease. At the time it had been observed that Americans appeared to have higher heart attack rates than people with poor nutrition living in countries that had been ravaged by the war.

Keyes drew the conclusion that the consumption of a lot of meat and dairy – in particular saturated fat – was related to high cholesterol and higher risk of heart disease. He also claimed that people eating low fat, more plant-based diets had low rates of heart disease.

Something people didn't know at the time was Keyes had manipulated the data. Actually, what he had done was "cherry pick" the data, only including data in his study that confirmed his hypothesis. He conveniently left out any data that contradicted it. He had in fact found cases where countries following low fat diets had higher rates of heart disease and some countries with more meat and fat-based diets had lower rates of heart disease. But since this wasn't discovered until much later, his study caught on and doctors readily accepted the claims.

From this, the modern view of diet that we've been living with for 50 years was born. By the end of the 1960s, the views that Keyes promoted were widely accepted by the medical establishment and the nutrition community. The food industry adapted fairly quickly, and by the 1980s people were eating special k cereal with skim milk for breakfast, and avoiding eggs and bacon, while also cutting way back on steaks and other red meat. Eggs were deemed to be so bad that they made the cover of Time magazine, with the viewpoint that eggs were dangerous and could lead to heart attack.

The Obesity Epidemic

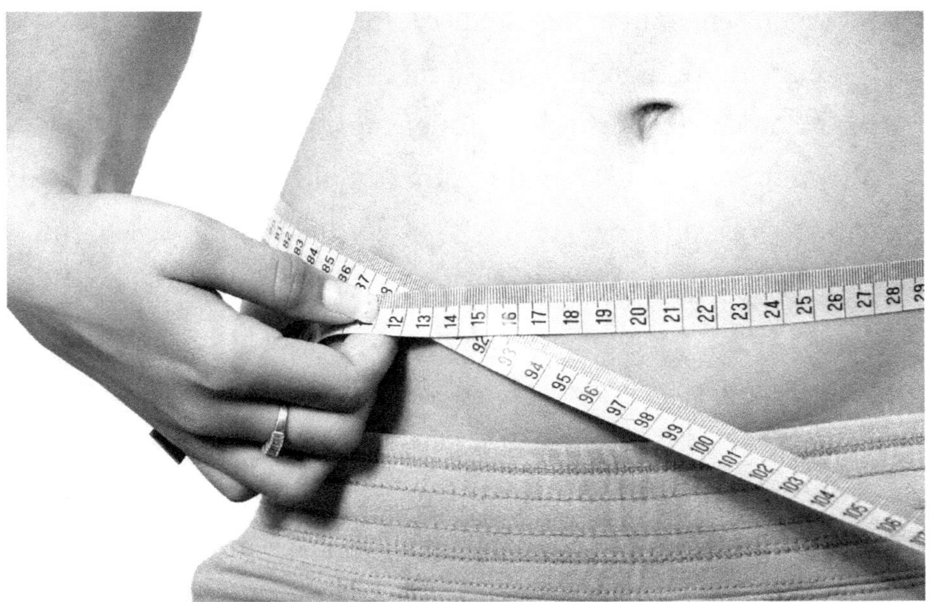

Oddly, something else was going on. It developed slowly, but insidiously. While people were supposedly eating healthier diets, people began gaining weight. As the 1990s turned into the new century, this trend began to catch fire and explode. It was as if people were becoming obese on an exponential curve, which starts out relatively slowly, and then suddenly takes off. Today, about 40% of Americans are so overweight that they are categorized as obese. This is a major problem of course, because obesity can lead to diabetes, heart attack, stroke, liver disease, and even cancer. In addition, people who are obese will have a much harder time getting around when they are older, and they are more likely to develop arthritis. Women are slightly more likely to be obese and men are slightly less likely to be obese. If we are just talking about people who are overweight and still at elevated risk for all the same health problems, more than 60% of adults are either overweight or obese. Some 30% of children under the age of 18 are overweight or obese, something that would have been unheard of 30, 40, or 50 years ago.

Doctors and the fitness/nutrition establishment look at this and come out with the same old advice. People need to watch their calories and exercise more. The view seems to be that people have some kind of character flaw, but the truth is that people have tried to follow the advice in large numbers. And yet, they can't seem to lose weight. What's going on?

Low Carb Dieting, and Keto Returns

In the early 1960s, a counter-trend was already in development, but it would take years before it finally became widespread among the public. A cardiologist named Dr. Atkins was working with his patients when he began noticing that patients eating fewer carbohydrates began losing weight and improving their health. After observing this he began putting his patients on a diet that he designed, which was low carb and high in fat and protein. This later became the basis of the Atkins diet, which he first popularized in a paperback book that came out in the early 1970s. But it really didn't catch fire until the mid to late 1990s.

The Atkins diet bears some similarity to the keto diet, but it allows the consumption of a lot more protein. It is also phased, rather than permanent so that over time people are allowed to consume more carbohydrates, but they are never going to be eating as many carbs as people do following the standard American diet. Nonetheless, people following the original Atkins diet had amazing results, losing large amounts of weight rapidly.

The same old complaints from skeptics that we hear now became widespread back then. People complained that eating low carb would hurt your kidneys because you were getting too much protein. They also claimed that people were losing "water weight", even when people were losing 30, 40, and 50 pounds. It was also claimed it was dangerous, possibly leading to heart attack and stroke, even though there wasn't any actual evidence of this.

At about the same time, people began rediscovering the ketogenic diet. But once again, it wasn't applied to weight loss but continued to be used for the purposes of treating epilepsy. This time the focus was almost entirely on childhood epilepsy. Due to some popularization in the mainstream press and the ability of people to share information on the now budding internet, the use of the ketogenic diet to manage epilepsy began gaining steam. But it would remain the background as far as being used for a diet to promote weight loss for many more years.

The Atkins diet remained fairly popular after the year 2000, but unfortunately Dr. Atkins had an accident slipping on the ice and hit his dead, and he died from internal bleeding. Even in death, the skeptics tried to make up stories that he had actually had a heart attack and that it was found that his arteries were clogged. None of that was true, but the worst thing about his death was that the Atkins diet and the organization promoting it was taken over by a group of people that believed in low carb dieting, but they were also heavily influenced by the erroneous viewpoint that fat is bad for you. So, the diet was modified somewhat, and after that it began losing popularity.

The Sugar Connection

In the 2000s, an author named Gary Taubes wrote a breakthrough book called *Why We Get Fat*. The book was a tour de force of nutrition, and it explained how sugar and carbohydrates make people gain weight. It also explained why fat was not harmful and explained how digestion works for the general public. So, it turned out that the high-carbohydrate way of eating that now permeated American society was largely responsible for the obesity epidemic we were now in the midst of. Besides eating lots of carbs in the form of bread and pasta, people consumed lots of sugar, often in the form of junk foods but also as fruit juice that they were led to believe was healthy.

At about this same time, the keto diet began coming back into the mainstream, but this time people began using it lose weight.

It turns out that you can power your body on fat, and this was the connection between fasting and the ketogenic diet that doctors had found decades earlier when using it to treat epilepsy. This is something that we will revisit in chapter seven, but what happens to your body, provided that you fast long enough, is your body switches from burning sugar to burning fat for energy. This process is known as ketosis. It turns out that despite our focus on using carbohydrates for energy, that the body is quite well adapted to burning fat for fuel. If your body can do it while fasting, and it does that naturally without any effort, then it makes sense to believe that if you consume a diet that is low in carbohydrates your body will be able to use fat for fuel under those circumstances as well. In the next chapter we will discuss how this works in detail.

Keto Diet and Weight Loss

The magic of the keto diet happens when your body adapts to a fat burning state. When you try doing this the first time, it's not something that happens instantly but rather over the course of a few days. In the fat burning state, your body can burn fat that you eat but it also burns the fat on your body. Under supposed normal circumstances when you are eating a diet that contains significant amounts of carbohydrates, when you are fasting, which is just going several hours without food (it doesn't have to be anything extreme), the body is capable of switching to a fat burning mode and it uses your own body fat for energy. However, if you are in a perpetual state of fat burning because you eat lots of fat and don't eat carbohydrates in large amounts, you will also be continually burning your body fat and switch in between burning dietary body fat and your own body fat quite readily. This leads to rapid and sustainable weight loss. In the next chapter we will explore how this works in detail.

Chapter 2: How Keto Works

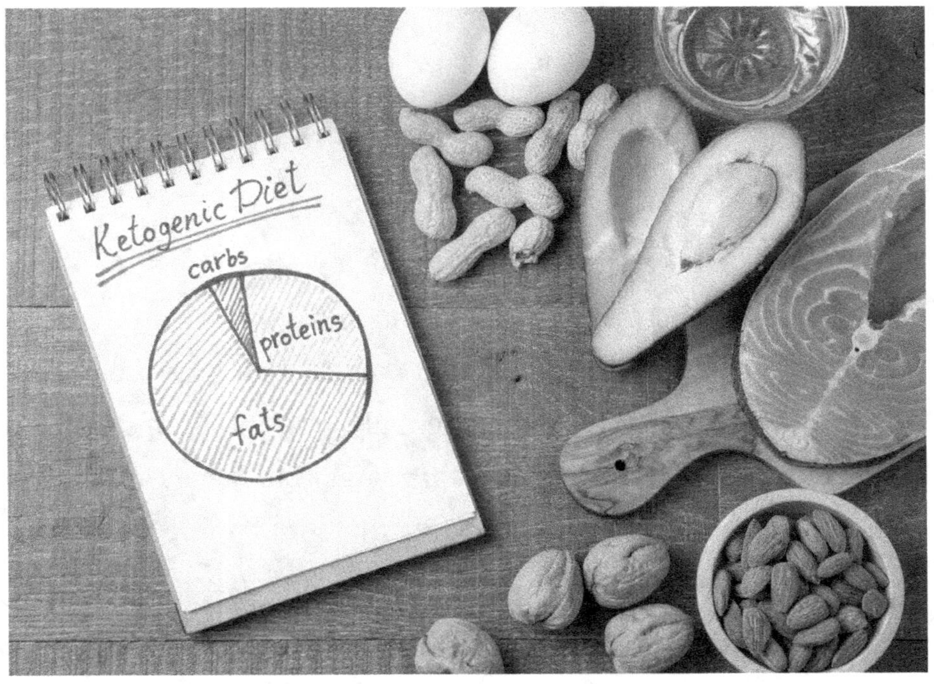

Now that we've set the stage for the keto diet it's time to explore how it works. First, we'll begin by explaining how the body gets energy from carbohydrates, which is something that most of us have been doing all of our lives until we discovered the keto diet. Then we'll explain what happens when you stop eating carbohydrates and how the body adapts. Once you understand this, you are going to understand why the keto diet can literally prevent or even reverse type 2 diabetes, and you'll also understand how consuming carbohydrates can cause type 2 diabetes. Then we will talk about the benefits of keto related to several diseases and the side effects of keto that you may encounter early on while following the diet.

Ketosis is a state when the body is burning fat for energy rather than sugar. A keto diet can induce ketosis without having to fast.

Digestion of Carbohydrates

Let's explore what happens when you digest carbohydrates. The first thing that happens is that your body begins breaking them down. Carbohydrates are actually long chains of sugar molecules, but unless the individual sugar molecules are split apart, your body can't use them. So, the initial phase of digestion is to break down the carbohydrate molecules that were in the bread, pasta, rice, or whatever else you ate into the individual sugar molecules. These are then released into the blood stream. These individual sugar molecules are called glucose.

When your blood sugar begins to rise, this triggers your pancreas. This is a digestive organ that lies behind your stomach on the left side of your body. Most people don't think much about their pancreas, and often people only think about it when they become ill because something has gone wrong with it, either from diabetes or pancreatic cancer. The pancreas plays a central role in digestion, releasing many digestive enzymes that help break down starches, proteins, and fats, and also by releasing hormones that basically define the digestive state of the body.

One of those hormones is insulin. You may have heard of it in the context of diabetes. Many diabetics need to inject insulin before they eat to help them derive energy from the carbohydrates in their diet. This is because either their pancreas doesn't make enough insulin any more or the body has become so desensitized to insulin that large amounts of it are required in order to digest foods and get the energy from them.

Insulin has several jobs that it has to accomplish that are related to digestion and the extraction and storage of energy from food. The first job that insulin has is getting the cells in your body to take up the glucose that is flowing around in your blood. The cells can use glucose to satisfy their energy needs, but it has to get inside the cell before they can use it. It takes insulin to make this happen. Many medical professionals use a lock and key analogy to explain how this works. You can think of the cell as having a locked door through which the glucose must pass in order to get inside the cell. Insulin provides the key that will open the door.

Unfortunately, many people become insulin resistant. That is, for a given amount of insulin in the blood stream, the cells don't respond and won't take up the glucose. So, if you imagine that originally it took one insulin molecule to get a cell to take up a molecule of glucose, maybe when a person hits age 25, now it's two insulin molecules. Then by the time they are 35 it's three insulin molecules that the cell needs before it takes up that glucose molecule.

These numbers aren't necessarily realistic but they serve to illustrate the point. As many of us age, we need more and more insulin in order to put that glucose to use. People who are experiencing this might not feel quite right, they will be fatigued more than normal because their body isn't completely using up the glucose that is coming from their diets.

This is something that you can measure as well. If you are insulin resistant, your blood glucose level is going to go higher than normal because your cells are not as able to use the glucose as the cells in a person who is "normal". Yes – I am putting that in quotes – consider the viewpoint that maybe our bodies aren't meant to be powered by carbohydrates, but instead we are meant to be powered by fat. If that's the case, then maybe there isn't really something wrong with people who are not so good at processing sugar after digesting it.

So, if you are able to digest sugar without issues, your blood sugar will rise to maybe 140 mg/dL two hours after eating. Someone who is diabetic or pre-diabetic will see their blood sugars rise to 180 mg/dL or even over 200 mg/dL. Their blood sugar goes higher and stays high for longer periods of time. This is simply the sugar that can't get into the cells where it could be used for energy. Eventually, a person will get to a point where their blood sugar is chronically elevated. In between meals or even in the morning after going hours without eating, they may have blood sugar levels that are as high as someone who isn't diabetic or pre-diabetic has after a meal.

Blood sugar above certain levels in your blood is not a good thing. Think about a sugary liquid. It's sticky and doesn't flow well. People who are diabetic can have a lot of sugar in their blood. In fact, diabetes was recognized in ancient India and they would test a person for diabetes by seeing if sugar ants were attracted to their blood and urine.

Sticky blood means that your body isn't able to get blood through the small capillaries in your body the way it should. Over time, this can start damaging your organs, like your kidneys. This in turn can lead to high blood pressure. The small blood vessels in your eye can become damaged, and eventually this can lead to blindness. Blood vessel damage can lead to erectile dysfunction and impotence. And finally, if someone with chronically high blood sugars gets an injury on their feet or lower legs, since blood flow through the small blood vessels is more restricted than normal, they will have problems with wound healing. If this isn't treated the wounds can become infected, and this can get so bad that amputation may become necessary.

Problems with blood glucose are at the root of many of the consequences of diabetes. Over time, blood vessel damage combined with high blood pressure will lead to heart disease and stroke. In fact, diabetics are at heightened risk for developing heart disease. Some estimates suggest that diabetics are four times as likely to have a heart attack as someone from the general population who is not diabetic. Diabetics are also at much higher risk than the general public for developing cancer. Doctors are now realizing that cancer too, is related to carbohydrate consumption.

Insulin helps make you fat

So, what happens to any glucose that your body can't use? Insulin plays a role here as well. First of all, your liver stores some glucose that can be used for energy when you need it or during an emergency. If the liver has any capacity to store more of it, insulin will prompt the liver to do so. The liver stores sugar by linking glucose molecules together in order to form starches that are called glycogen. These starchy molecules are broken down when the body is in a fasting state in order to provide energy. However, the capacity of this storage to provide energy is very limited, in many cases your liver can only keep blood sugar levels up for several hours.

That is something that we will use to our advantage on the keto diet.

Since the ability of the liver to store glucose is limited, and it's probably stored plenty in the past if you are regularly eating a carbohydrate-based diet, that sugar has to go somewhere. What happens now is that the liver will assemble the molecules into fats. They are then released into the blood stream. Insulin then signals your fat cells to take them up, so that they can store some more fat. So that is basically why people get fat, you have some excess glucose in your bloodstream that your body can't use for energy. Then insulin has the liver converting into fat and then it tells the fat cells to take it up. Your fat cells have a basically unlimited capacity to store fat. So, this is a situation that could be out of control.

What happens when digestion is over?

After insulin has done its job, as much as it is capable of doing, your body switches gears. Your pancreas makes another hormone that is called glucagon. Basically, this is the fasting hormone. So, any time that you are not consuming food, your body is in a fasting state once it gets done with digesting whatever food you most recently ate. As some people say the body can be in one of two states, a fed state and a fasted state. So, to understand what is going on, note that the fed state is dominated by the hormone insulin, which puts fat on the body, and the fasting state is dominated by the hormone glucagon.

The first thing that glucagon does is it will tell the liver to break down that stored sugar and release it into the blood stream. The first impulse of the body is to keep blood sugar levels high. And if you are living on a carbohydrate diet, this makes perfect sense.

But remember that the liver only has so much glycogen. When it runs out, glucagon stimulates your fat cells to release fat into the blood stream. Then it directs the liver to take up this fat, and break it down into molecules called ketones, and to release them into the blood stream.

So, glucagon is the hormone that takes fat off the body.

You can think of ketones as the fat equivalent to glucose. Your cells can burn ketones for energy. However, not all cells in your body can burn ketones. Red blood cells can't, for example.

Some cells in your kidneys can't burn ketones either. Your brain can burn ketones – if it couldn't children with epilepsy would not be able to use a keto diet to manage their symptoms. However, your brain needs sugar to power about 30% of it's energy needs. So, 70% of the brain's energy needs can be provided by fat through ketones.

Provided that you are not suffering from an illness and subject to hypoglycemia, your body is able to make sure that blood sugar levels are adequate to satisfy these narrowly tailored needs for sugar as fuel. This can be done through protein intake. Through a process called gluconeogenesis, the body can make sugar out of protein that you consume in your diet (or in extreme circumstances that we want to avoid – out of your own muscle tissue). Keep in mind however that the body's use of protein to make glucose is something that is restricted. Your body is not going to raise blood sugar from the consumption of protein. It makes just enough blood sugar out of the protein to make sure that the brain, red blood cells, and kidneys are getting the amount of blood sugar that is needed.

Otherwise, your body does perfectly well powered by fat. In fact, many scientists are actually arguing that this is the natural state of the body. Prehistoric humans, especially those that lived in ice aged Europe and Asia, basically survived on ketogenic diets. They ate high amounts of protein and animal fat, and only had small amounts of vegetables available. This is a situation that went on for hundreds of thousands of years, so it's quite possible that the human body is actually naturally adapted for fat burning.

Conventional science, at least until recently but still believed by many, claims that sugar burning is the natural state of the body, but it can use fat burning as an emergency backup. Maybe – things are the other way around. And maybe the natural state of the body is to burn fat for energy while using sugar as fuel only in emergencies. Like when it was hard to hunt down and kill a large animal.

Ketones

There are three ketones that can be produced. They are made by the liver from fat molecules. One of them is actually not usable and it's excreted in the breath and in urine. People just starting the keto diet will experience some bad breath as a result of this, but that is something that passes with time. The other two ketones can be used to generate energy for the body. This is done in the power factories inside your body's cells, in the mitochondria. They have different chemical pathways that can be used to generate energy that they provide for the cell. When sugar is present, the fat burning pathway is blocked. But when sugar is in short supply, the fat burning pathway is available, and your body will then use fat for energy production. Let's summarize what we know.

So now you know why people get fat. It's the sugar, stupid! People eat carbohydrates – of any kind – and these are broken down into glucose molecules (sugar) by the digestive system. Insulin tries to get your cells to take it up and use it for energy. Any left over glucose is sent to the liver where it can be stored up to a certain amount, or insulin prompts the liver to make fat molecules out of it which are then released to the blood stream, then insulin gets your fat cells to take it up and store it. Now you're fat!

Glucagon is the opposite hormone. It drives fat out of your fat cells and into the liver, where it's broken down into ketone bodies, which are then used by the body for energy. So, glucagon is a fat burning hormone. This is important to note, and we also need to reiterate that if you consume significant levels of carbohydrates with your meals, you are going to be releasing insulin, and not glucagon. So, a high fat meal that contains a lot of carbs is still going to contribute to you getting fatter. A high fat meal without carbs isn't going to contribute to you getting fatter, because in that case, glucagon is going to be in control and insulin levels will be low. You will be in a fasting state as far as the hormones in your body are concerned.

When your body is in ketosis, it will have ketones in the blood. There are home test kits available to check this if you want to do so. They come in three basic types. You can use urine test strips, a breath test, or a small device that will test your blood for the presence of ketones. The latter is probably the best method to use. The desired range for ketosis is 0.5-3 mmol/L.

It's important to distinguish ketosis from ketoacidosis. Unfortunately, many in the medical and nutritional community don't do so, and they try to scare people away from the keto diet by mixing up the two. Let's get this straight – ketosis is not the same as ketoacidosis at all. Ketosis is a perfectly normal state of the body when you are not consuming significant levels of carbohydrates. Ketoacidosis is a condition that happens in untreated diabetics. This occurs when they are not able to produce enough insulin and they have very high blood sugar levels, that can be 300 mg/dL or higher. The body produces ketones as an emergency response to these very high and abnormal blood sugar levels and the low insulin levels. Symptoms include frequent urination, excessive thirst, vomiting, confusion, and shortness of breath.

Eating a keto diet is never going to cause ketoacidosis. It just doesn't do it, and ketoacidosis is associated with very high blood sugar levels. If you are not an untreated diabetic and you are following the ketogenic diet, you are not going to have high blood sugar levels. In fact, people on the ketogenic diet will see their blood sugar levels drop. So, if anyone is telling you that the keto diet causes this condition, you know that they are not to be believed.

If you are still worried about it, you can get an all-in-one meter that will test your blood sugar and ketone level simultaneously. These are available on Amazon and can be helpful for those on the keto diet. That way you can put your mind at ease making sure that your blood sugars are in normal ranges and that your ketones are not at excessive levels.

The Main Benefits of Keto

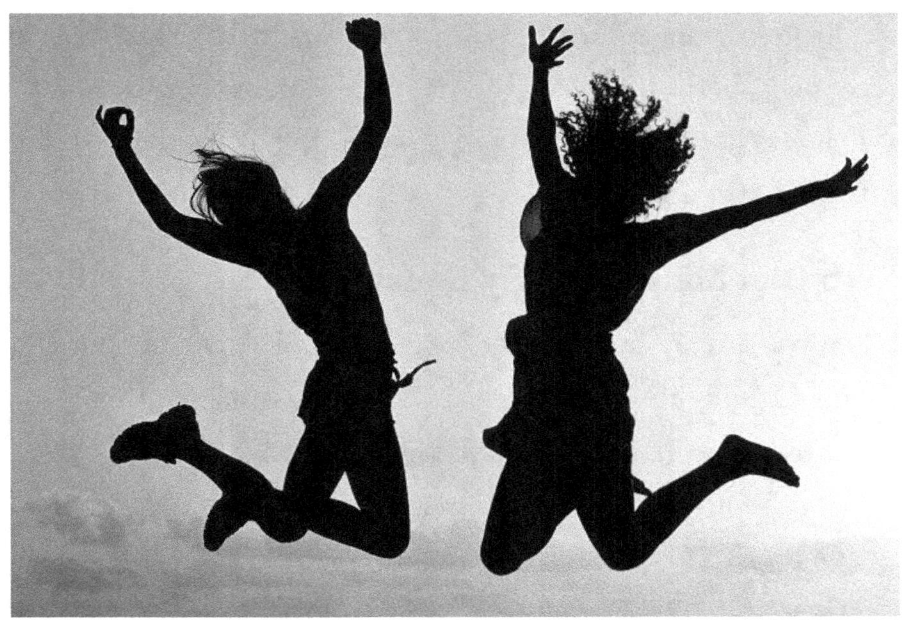

The keto diet has many benefits for the body. There is mounting evidence that although the brain does need to get about 30% of its energy needs met by blood sugar, its better off getting the rest from ketones. Getting your energy from ketones also helps keep your energy levels steady. Something that comes to mind is how you can quickly burn off a meal based on simple carbohydrates. Think if you just ate a muffin or a bagel for breakfast (or worse a donut). A couple of hours later chances are you're going to be hungry. Some people are going to find that they are super hungry, even famished, after eating a muffin or bagel without anything else. You might experience the same phenomenon eating Chinese food. Some Chinese restaurants use a lot of sugar in their sauces, and so you have a meal with a lot of sugar-laden sauce, mostly vegetables, and white rice. And the meal won't stay with you. Two hours later, you're going to be super hungry, almost as if you had never eaten.

Keto Diet Means Steady Energy Levels

When you are on the keto diet, if you are getting enough fat you are never going to experience this. The most amazing thing about the keto diet is how satisfying a meal that contains a lot of fat without carbohydrates is going to be. Let's explore the reason that this is the case.

When you eat a meal that is heavy in simple carbs, such as a plain muffin with nothing else, here is what happens. As the muffin is digested, it's broken down into glucose. That glucose is then released into the blood stream and your insulin levels shoot up. If you are not insulin resistant, then your cells are going to take up as much of the glucose that you need, and insulin is going to push the rest of the glucose that is above the background level of blood sugar into the liver where it's converted into fat, and then the insulin will cause the fat cells to take it up. This process happens rather quickly. Someone without diabetes is going to see their blood sugar quickly ramp up to a peak of about 140 mg/dL and drop back down to 110 mg/dL or less. The sugar is quickly used in the cells for energy, and after that they have nothing. The rise and fall of blood sugar levels can make you feel weak and irritable or fatigued.

Now suppose that you are on the keto diet and you eat an avocado, an egg, and a couple of strips of fatty bacon for breakfast. First of all, your body is already in a fasted state and so you aren't changing a thing by eating. Insulin levels are very low, at background levels, and your bloodstream has more glucagon, the fat burning hormone. While you were sleeping, your body was already producing ketones from your body fat.

So, when you eat this meal which contains hardly any carbohydrates at all, your body is just going to continue along in the state that it's already in. The fat in the meal will be broken down into ketones and used for fuel. Remember – you're already in a ketone burning state, and so nothing really changes. Over the course of the day the fat from the meal is gradually burned for fuel, but there is no rising and falling of blood sugar levels. Your body is in a steady-state, for all intents and purposes.

Keep in mind that in the beginning, it's going to take time to adjust to keto. The reason is that your body has stored sugars in your liver called glycogen. When you are just starting out, you need to burn off the glycogen before your body actually adapts to ketosis. If you have never engaged in fasting and have been eating a standard American diet that contains a large amount of carbohydrates, you are going to find that it takes time to do this. It can take as long as a few days.

However, once your body has burned off the glycogen, it will begin adapting to the fat burning state.

Massive Weight Loss

The second benefit of keto is the main reason that people are adopting this diet. That is, you are going to have rapid and sustainable weight loss. One of the criticisms of keto by those who are truly ignorant about the diet is that you are only losing "water weight". The fact is, for the first week that is going to be true! You would be surprised how much water is used to store glycogen in your liver. Each molecule of the start glycogen is bound to four molecules of water. So, when you are burning off the glycogen, as the body breaks it down into blood sugar to use, you are going to be releasing a lot of water.

However, that process is only going to last for a few days to maybe a week. Once your body has gotten the glycogen level down to a minimum it's going to be burning fat for energy, which means that you're going to be losing weight from burning fat, not from losing water weight. So, the myth does have a grain of truth to it, but saying that you are only losing water weight is something that can only be applied to someone who only follows the keto diet for a week or less. If you stay on the keto diet over the long term, you are going to be burning fat, not "water weight".

It's important to note that for some people the loss of weight and body fat is not going to be steady. It may happen in spurts. For this reason, you should not be weighing yourself constantly. Don't weigh yourself every single day, try weighing yourself every 3 days or even just once a week. You might also focus on other metrics like measuring your waistline, rather than just focusing on your weight – because it's really loss of body fat that is the most important metric. If you are working out while following a keto diet you might find that you are putting on more muscle mass at the same time that you are losing fat, and so at times your weight may not go down, but you are still losing body fat.

Second weight can fluctuate day to day, but still be heading on a downward trend. Have you ever looked at stock market charts? If you do, you will see that they are all jittery, but they can be following a trend up or down even though over the short term, they bounce up and down a lot. For some people, their weight will do the same thing. So weighing yourself every single day will give you a distorted picture because it might go up a pound or two in a single day, but that might have no meaning at all over the course of a week, where you might have a net weight loss of three or four pounds.

Weighing yourself daily can cause you to get down if there are not apparent results. That is another reason to avoid doing it. I strongly recommend that you only weight yourself every three days at the most. If you are not making progress over the course of a week, then you might want to take a closer look at your diet and try to figure out what you are doing wrong.

Before I continue, we need to return to the issue of glycogen in your liver and the loss of water weight. This is a reason that it's important not to cheat on the keto diet. Let's think about what happens if you take a day off once a week. If you do that, after having spent three days burning off the glycogen in your liver, and then a few days burning fat, what is going to happen? First of all, on your cheat day your body is going to put some of that fat back on because you are consuming sugars. Second, your body is going to restock your liver. That means that the next day when you get back on your diet, you're going to have to spend time burning off the glycogen again. It's true that you are not going to have as much as you did when first starting out, because before you literally had years worth of glycogen stored up – but having a cheat day is going to set you back. So, the first day or two of returning to the diet, you're going to be burning the sugar stored in the liver and losing water weight.

Many people who follow the keto diet will experience a lot of initial weight loss, but then they will plateau. Don't get discouraged if this happens. Often, the weight loss will suddenly resume on its own. If you find that you are having an intractable problem, you might look at the ratios of fat and protein in your diet, and eat more fat and less protein. The rule of the keto diet is to eat fat to lose fat. While protein is not a problem for a lot of people, some are more sensitive to it and might need to restrict their protein intake.

Heightened Mental Clarity

Remember that the brain does better on the ketogenic diet. This was first demonstrated when it was used to treat epileptic children. At that time, they did studies beyond just looking at the seizures and found that the children were more focused and attentive, doing better at school. Since then more studies have found the same results, and there are also countless testimonials indicating that people simply feel better mentally with an increased ability to focus and think clearly when they are on the keto diet. Scientists are not sure why this is the case, but the results are clear, when its able to burn fat for fuel the brain does better. Its also possible that having a high fat diet helps the brain keep the myelin sheaths around the nerve cells intact, leading to better transmission of signals. If you don't know anything about the physiology of the brain, your brain cells have a part that could be loosely described as an electrical transmission line. And just like transmission lines in electrical systems, they work a lot better when the insulation is good.

Regardless of what causes it, the results are clear. People report that their memory improves, they are able to focus and pay attention better, and they have more overall mental clarity.

This is another one of those things that takes time to develop as your body adjusts to the keto diet. So, don't be discouraged if you don't find yourself with better mental clarity in the first few weeks. In fact, during the transition process you might find yourself experiencing mental fog instead. But as we'll see later that is a temporary effect that can be dealt with by some simple adjustments, and over time it's going to reverse. If the theory about the insulation of the brain cells is correct, that process probably takes time, your body would actually have to work on that.

Although it's not completely clear yet, a keto diet may have a positive impact on other neurological conditions. For example, it might help with MS and Parkinson's disease, and could possibly help reduce the risk and impact of Alzheimer's disease. We don't want to claim it's a cure all for neurological conditions, more research is needed. But the preliminary results are enticing.

Improves Heart Health

If you recall, the modern American diet, including that recommended by the USDA, became a low-fat diet as a result of some misguided studies linking cholesterol and saturated fat to heart disease. One of the surprising and welcome benefits of the keto diet is that it actually appears to reduce the risks of heart disease.

This is one thing that you are going to hear the naysayers harping on – they are going to tell you that following a keto diet over the long-term is a risky proposition when it comes to your heart health. However, the fact is they are completely wrong.

First let's get the saturated fat issue out of the way. For decades, the medical establishment accepted the claim that saturated fat increased heart disease risk. This connection largely came about because the consumption of saturated fat is directly related to your cholesterol level. In short, one of the things your body does with saturated fat is it makes cholesterol out of it. But as we will see below, things are not as simple as they first appear.

Your body needs cholesterol. It's used to make the "sex hormones" testosterone and estrogen. It's also a component of every cell wall in your body. It's also used to make a natural supply of vitamin D when your skin is exposed to sunlight, and research is showing that low vitamin D levels are directly connected to increased risk of several illnesses, including respiratory infections and cancer. Low vitamin D levels can even increase your risk of death from conditions like pneumonia and severe strains of flu.

So, cholesterol is not a completely evil molecule, even though we've had that notion shoved down our throats since the 1970s. It's an essential component of bodily functioning.

Very low levels of cholesterol have also been tied to health problems. In fact, people with very low cholesterol levels have higher risk of death from all causes. Very low levels of cholesterol are tied to increased risk of cancer, and even dementia.

Supposedly, the healthy level of total cholesterol is 200 mg/dL or less. But are you aware that half of all first-time heart attack victims have cholesterol levels that are below 200? That seems to indicate that the overall or total cholesterol level only tells a small part of the story – and we are going to see that in fact, that is the case.

But let's return to saturated fat. The primary source of saturated fat is from animal products like beef and chicken skin. However, it's also presents in coconut and it's also found in smaller amounts in plant oils like olive oil. We know that saturated fat intake does raise your cholesterol level. But is it really connected with increase heart attack risk?

Since 2010, there have been multiple large-scale studies that have shown that there is no link, whatsoever, between saturated fat intake and heart disease risk. The connection between the two simply isn't there. At worse, saturated fat intake is something that could be considered to be neutral, that is it has no impact one way or another. However, the reality is saturated fat intake, if you are not consuming significant amounts of carbohydrates, is actually beneficial. It can actually reduce your risk of heart disease for many reasons.

Let's see why. The first reason that saturated fat can reduce your risk of heart disease and stroke is that you're going to be losing weight – and weight gain is directly associated with increased risk of cardiovascular disease. Second, if you are following a keto diet, the saturated fat you're consuming that is used for fuel means that you are either going to massively reduce your risk of getting diabetes, or possibly reverse diabetes if you already have it. Diabetics are up to four times as likely to have a heart attack as a member of the general population.

But if we dig deeper, there are more reasons why eating fat rather than carbohydrates, including saturated fat, is going to reduce your risk of heart disease and stroke. To understand why, we need to take a look at "blood fats" and cholesterol in more detail.

You probably know that your body has good and bad cholesterol. The good cholesterol is called HDL cholesterol. This type of cholesterol actually keeps the bloodstream clean of excess fat and cholesterol. It also keeps the walls of your arteries clean and can remove bad cholesterol that is stuck to your artery walls, reducing the risk of having a heart attack or stroke, because this reduces the risk of having a clot form. So, people with higher HDL cholesterol levels are at lower risk of heart attack and stroke. The lowest level of HDL that is deemed acceptable is 40 mg/dL. If your HDL is below this level, you are at elevated risk for having a heart attack or stroke. A number above 50 mg/dL is deemed healthy.

In some people, consumption of a high fat and low carbohydrate diet can lead to improved HDL levels. This may not happen for you, but as we'll see even if your HDL level doesn't increase, eating a high-fat and low-carb diet will have other impacts that are going to significantly decrease your risk. Some recent studies have shown that people that are able to stick to a ketogenic diet for a significant amount of time will see their HDL levels increase.

Bad cholesterol is called LDL cholesterol. It turns out that the form your bad cholesterol takes depends on what you eat. Bad cholesterol can be small and dense, or it can be larger and "light and fluffy" as some people put it. When its larger and light and fluffy, bad cholesterol flows through your bloodstream without doing much if any damage. So, in other words, it becomes harmless, rather than being "bad cholesterol".

Contrast this with small and dense LDL cholesterol molecules. These are truly bad cholesterol. The reason is, since they are small and dense, they can actually stick to artery walls. This can cause inflammation. That is a normal process that happens when injury occurs. Think about when you get a cut, and it becomes swollen and red. That happens as a result of your immune system trying to repair the damage. The same thing basically happens inside your arteries, but unfortunately the process can be damaging. In an effort to deal with the stuck LDL cholesterol molecules, clots are formed inside your arteries, and over time they can lead to partial blockages or artery narrowing, or become unstable and break off, causing a heart attack or stroke. In fact, a measure of inflammation can give you your risk of heart attack. This is done by measuring C-Reactive Protein, or CRP. This is an inflammation marker that is directly related to the amount of inflammation in your cardiovascular system.

Now the question becomes what causes LDL cholesterol to be small and dense? It turns out that a diet high in carbohydrates is the culprit. If you eat a diet that is high in fat while seriously restricting your carbohydrate intake, your LDL cholesterol molecules are going to become larger, and light and fluffy. This is going to reduce your heart disease and stroke risk.

Now let's take a look at triglycerides, which are a type of blood fat. Doctors didn't pay much attention to triglycerides in the past, in fact after the Ancel Keyes studies and for decades afterwards, they were completely ignored as far as heart disease and stroke risk were concerned. But guess what – your blood triglyceride level plays a direct role in your risk of developing heart disease and stroke.

In fact, the ratio of triglycerides to HDL cholesterol is the best measure of heart disease risk that there is, aside from direct scanning techniques like an echocardiogram or calcium CT scan.

If the ratio is 3.0 or greater, your risk of having a heart attack or stroke is much higher. If your ratio of triglycerides to HDL cholesterol is lower than 3.0, then your risk of heart attack or stroke is reduced. The closer to 1.0 it is, the lower your risk. If its 2.0 or lower, you are at very low risk of heart disease.

So how do you lower your triglycerides? One way to do it is to eat a lot of fish. This is why fish consumption is generally associated with lower risk of heart disease.

Another way to do it – is to follow a ketogenic diet. It turns out that high triglyceride levels can actually be caused by carbohydrate consumption. Unfortunately, there is a lot of misinformation out there when it comes to triglycerides, so it's important to correct that right now.

In the olden days, when none of this was understood, since triglycerides are a type of fat, the medical establishment latched onto the completely unproven idea that high levels of triglycerides in the bloodstream were caused by eating fat. In fact, many still believe this idea, even though it's been disproven. You can even see this falsehood still being promoted on websites associated with major medical institutions.

The thing is, there have been well designed studies on triglycerides to determine what causes them to rise. One recent study had participants increase their consumption of sugar by drinking large amounts of orange juice. The shocking result of this study wasn't that it causes increased levels of triglycerides – it certainly did – but rather how quickly the triglyceride levels rose. Eating a lot of sugar just over a few weeks will cause your triglyceride levels to increase. It might even happen nearly instantly.

To summarize – eating carbohydrates in large amounts, especially sugar – is what causes high triglycerides.

Second, you won't be surprised to hear this – following a ketogenic diet causes triglyceride levels to drop. This has been proven in studies and you will also find lots of personal accounts stating this result. As many people say, following a low carbohydrate diet will make your triglycerides drop like a rock. It's the opposite situation compared to drinking large amounts of orange juice, something proven to make triglyceride levels go sky-high. So, it shouldn't be surprising that one of the easiest ways to lower your triglyceride levels is to follow a ketogenic diet.

Another factor that is associated with heart disease is a large amount of abdominal fat. For some reason, fat piled around the organs in your abdomen is particularly risk when it comes to the risk of heart disease. It turns out that one of the many benefits of the ketogenic diet is that as a part of your overall weight loss, it seems to be particularly effective at reducing abdominal fat. That's just one more way that a ketogenic diet is going to make you more heart healthy.

So far, we've seen that a ketogenic diet is going to make your LDL cholesterol larger, light and fluffy, therefore reducing the risk that it will become lodged into your artery walls, leading to the formation of dangerous blood clots. Second, we've seen that a ketogenic diet is going to significantly decrease your triglycerides, and it might help to raise your HDL levels, thereby improving the ratio of triglycerides to HDL and reducing your cardiovascular disease risk significantly. Then we found out that a ketogenic diet reduces abdominal body fat. But there is one more way that a ketogenic diet reduces the risk of heart disease.

It does this by stabilizing your blood sugars. High blood sugar levels damage your blood vessels, and this can lead to heart disease down the road. In particular, blood sugar spikes seem to be related to the damaged caused in your blood vessels. If you are following a ketogenic diet, over time you are going to find that your blood sugar levels are reduced on average – but more importantly nobody on a ketogenic diet ever has a blood sugar spike. So, by following a ketogenic diet you are going to stop doing damage to your arteries that can occur from high blood sugars.

These results are paradoxical, only if you subscribe to the false notions that have plagued the medical and nutritional establishments over the past 50 years. They've been living a lie, promoting the idea that fat is bad for you and that a high fat diet not only makes you fat, but that it causes heart disease and stroke. The data are coming in and the reality is that a high fat diet does neither if you reduce your intake of carbohydrates.

Lower Blood Pressure

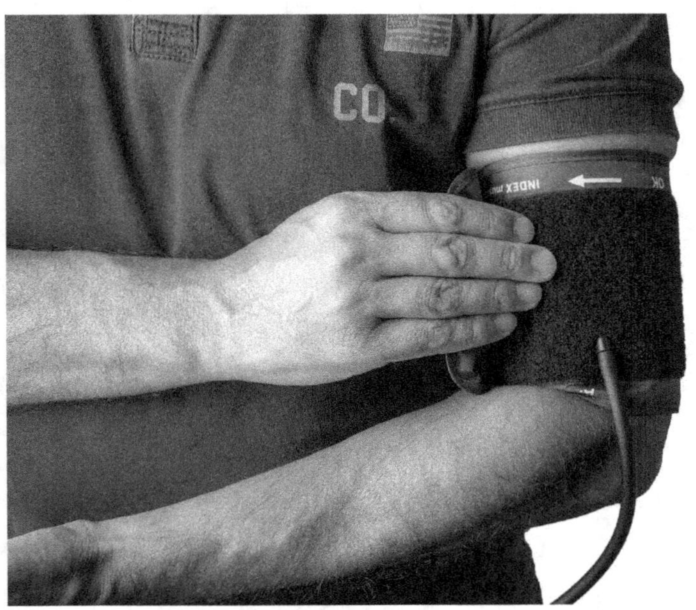

Blood pressure is another risk factor when it comes to heart disease and stroke, and it's also a risk factor for kidney disease. High blood pressure is called the "silent killer" because until the end stages of the disease, it causes no symptoms. Luckily in the modern era, high blood pressure can be managed with medications. But it turns out that the ketogenic diet will help control blood pressure in some people.

There are many possible causes of high blood pressure, but in most cases, doctors won't be able to figure out a cause. However, high insulin levels, in particular if you have chronically high insulin levels, can lead to high blood pressure. When you start following a ketogenic diet, your insulin levels are going to drop because you don't need insulin nearly as much as you used to. This isn't going to work with everyone, but some people are going to find that their blood pressure levels decrease as a result when they start the ketogenic diet. If you are on high blood pressure medications, you might want to carefully monitor your blood pressure when you start a ketogenic diet, because you may need to adjust your medications as a result. In fact, some people are able to get off their blood pressure medications when they are following a ketogenic diet. Keep in mind that this happens in some cases and not others. Unfortunately, some people may have high blood pressure levels for many different genetic or family history reasons, and so following a ketogenic diet may not reduce their blood pressure levels, or reduce them enough so that they can get off their medications. You will just have to see what happens in your particular situation if you are currently on blood pressure medications.

Another way that the ketogenic diet can help some people with blood pressure comes simply from the fact that you are going to be losing weight. Being overweight, by itself, seems to increase the risk of having high blood pressure. So, by losing weight on the keto diet, you can cut your risk of developing high blood pressure. And if you have high blood pressure now and it's a result of you being overweight or obese, losing a significant amount of weight is probably going to help you reset your blood pressure to healthy levels.

Reduced Cancer Risk

A few years after doctors began using the ketogenic diet in order to treat epilepsy, a scientist in Germany named Otto Warburg began doing experiments with cancer. He discovered that most cancer cells need to have sugar to survive. This fact languished in obscurity for many years, but over the past 20 years it's gained renewed interest. The evidence not only indicates that cancer cells (of most types) can't survive without sugar, but that consuming a high-fat and low carbohydrate diet can actually stop cancer in its tracks, and may even be able to cure it.

Many people may not realize this, but high blood sugar levels are associated with the development of many cancers, and diabetics that are untreated are at twice the risk of developing cancer. Colon cancer and pancreatic cancer seem to be closely associated with high blood sugar levels.

Although your body is always going to maintain your blood sugar levels within a narrow range, even while following a ketogenic diet, it appears that if blood sugar levels are below a certain value your risk of developing cancer drops substantially. If you are getting your energy from ketones this also lowers the risk.

Note that sugar probably doesn't cause cancer, there are many causes of cancer. What sugar does is it helps cancer grow and become a disease that threatens the body. Sugar is literally poison when viewed in this way, at least when we think about consuming large amounts of it.

Several scientists doing fundamental research on cancer not only verified the discoveries of Warburg, which are now known as the Warburg effect, but they have discovered that the energy machines in cancer cells – the mitochondria – are defective. While normal mitochondria are able to produce energy using sugar or fat, mitochondria in most types of cancer cells must have sugar to produce energy, and they cannot produce energy from fat. One result of this is that many of them will die off if you are not consuming high levels of carbohydrates.

Among the scientists that are supportive of the connection between sugar and cancer is the discoverer of DNA himself – James Watson. According to a New York Times article on the topic, although he is not diabetic, Watson believes in this idea so strongly that he takes metformin to keep his blood sugar levels low. In fact, there are studies showing that taking metformin reduces the risk of cancer among diabetes patients significantly. But you don't need to take metformin – something that comes with side effects as all drugs do – you can reduce your risk significantly just by following a ketogenic diet.

Scientists are only in the early stages of investigating the use of a ketogenic diet with actual cancer patients, but the time to deal with this is before you get cancer in the first place. Sticking to the ketogenic diet if you do get cancer will be vitally important to benefit from these effects.

However, tests using animals have definitely proven that there are practical results that follow from a low-carb diet when it comes to cancer. In one study, scientists purposely gave mice breast cancer and some other types of cancers. They had a control group that ate the standard diet for mice, which is a high-carbohydrate diet. Then they fed other groups of mice two low carb diets, one limited carbohydrate intake to 15% of total calories, and another limited it to 8-10% of total calories. Note that this diet was actually a high protein diet and not a keto diet, although in part it made up for the lost calories from carbohydrates by increasing the amount of fat in the diet.

They found that even the 15% diet led to much better results than a normal diet with respect to cancer. The extent that the cancer developed was significantly reduced, with smaller tumors and less metastasis (spread of the cancer to other organs). However, the 8-10% level of carbohydrate intake produced the best results. The mice on the low carb diet were able to live a normal lifespan, even though they had cancer. So, in many cases the result isn't necessarily that the cancer was completely cured, but rather that the mice were able to live out their entire lives with the cancer because its development was arrested.

These results show that it's the limitation of carbohydrates that is the primary factor, and that having a high protein intake isn't going to promote cancer growth. However, fundamental research shows that the keto diet, which has reduced protein intake as well, leads to better results.

One interesting application of this research is at the ketupat sanctuary. Although they are working with small numbers so far, they have had dramatic results curing or arresting cancer in dogs. In many cases, very advanced cases of cancer have been cured. Hemangiosarcoma is a cancer of blood vessels that is relatively common in dogs, and they have found that a ketogenic diet was able to completely eliminate all evidence of tumors in some dogs that had metastatic disease that was very advanced when they arrived at the sanctuary. The dogs follow a very strict ketogenic diet that limits total carbohydrate intake to 5-8% of total calories and is very high fat. They also use hyperbaric oxygen therapy, which may help improve results. Keep in mind that this doesn't cure or reverse cancer in all cases, but it has done so for many of the dogs that have been put on the program.

Reduces Acne

Now we move from a very serious health concern to a more minor one, but it appears that the ketogenic diet is able to reduce the incidence of acne. This is because in many cases, acne is a results of blood sugar levels. By keeping blood sugar levels consistently lower, the ketogenic diet is able to reduce the overall incidence of acne. Some have proposed that this is also a result of the populations of bacteria in your stomach and intestines. It turns out that what you eat is going to be directly correlated with the types of bacteria, because different bacteria digest different types of food. So, if you switch from a high carbohydrate to a high fat and low carbohydrate diet, the proportion of different types of bacteria in your gut is going to change. This may be indirectly related to the management of blood sugar levels and the development of acne, and studies are showing that the keto diet leads to better skin health.

Keto Side Effects

When you first start the ketogenic diet, you may develop certain side effects. These vary from person to person, and many people are able to adopt the keto diet without having any side effects at all, while other people are going to find that the keto diet causes a lot of problems in the first month. We will discuss dealing with these problems in detail in a later chapter, for now we will go over what these problems are that you might develop.

Changing from a diet that includes a lot of carbohydrates, and often a lot of accompanying high levels of dietary fiber, to one that is largely based on fat intake can be quite a shock to the body. Also, as we'll see later this can also require some adjustments to the consumption of minerals and certain vitamins.

The most common complaint that people have is that they are experiencing something known as the "keto flu". The keto flu is basically a state of low energy, where you feel constantly drained and fatigued. This is going to be something that happens as your body adjusts to the keto diet.

People who are not careful about what they are consuming may also develop kidney stones on the keto diet. In chapter 4, we will reveal some ways that you can reduce your risk for this unpleasant side effect, but note that the development of kidney stones on the keto diet is actually something that is relatively rare.

Some people might find that they are losing muscle mass on the keto diet. This will only happen if you consume levels of protein that are inadequate. In chapter 5, we will discuss the amounts of protein that your body needs and how to get adequate levels of protein while still consuming the right ratios of fat, protein, and carbohydrates.

Other people are going to develop problems related to digestion. The most common effect that occurs is constipation, but some people can actually develop diarrhea when their body is first exposed to a large amount of fat in the diet. We will discuss both of these issues in chapter 5.

Reducing heartburn

One interesting side effect of the keto diet that is a major benefit is that it reduces heart burn. Patients that have GERD have been proven to have improvements in symptoms after adopting a keto diet, and in fact other studies have shown that high levels of carbohydrate intake cause GERD to get worse. And as a matter of practicality, as you go on a keto diet and reduce your abdominal fat, it's going to help relieve heartburn and GERD because you will have less fat pushing down on your stomach and forcing stomach acid up into your esophagus.

Metabolic Syndrome

When people hit middle age, which might be defined as the age range of 40-65, many people develop a medical condition called metabolic syndrome. This condition isn't a disease in and of itself, but it is symptomatic of an inability to digest and manage carbohydrates in large amounts. Of course, many in the medical establishment don't discuss it in this way, because they don't want to admit that the high-carb and low-fat diets they've been advocating all these years are the cause of the problem. Let's cut to the chase – they are the cause of the problem.

So, what is metabolic syndrome? It's a cluster of symptoms that all stem from a lifetime of carbs. The first symptom of metabolic syndrome is a large belly. People with metabolic syndrome tend to put fat on in their abdominal area, and this increases their risk of developing cardiovascular disease.

This heightened risk is confirmed when you examine their blood lipids. You are going to find that people with abdominal fat in larger amounts tend have high triglycerides, high bad cholesterol, and low HDL cholesterol levels. The combination of these factors is a part of metabolic syndrome.

In addition, those with metabolic syndrome are going to have high blood pressure. They can also have high blood sugars.

Their blood sugar does not have to be at diabetic levels, but it will be higher than what is considered to be normal.

In short, metabolic syndrome is an end stage of a lifetime of eating carbohydrates and it might have been made worse by failing to get enough exercise or improperly managing stress. But metabolic syndrome isn't the end state, it's actually a precursor to the development of many serious diseases. People with metabolic syndrome are at much higher risk of developing diabetes in the coming years. In addition, they are at much higher risk of developing heart disease or stroke, and their risk of cancer is elevated in many cases.

One of the leading benefits of the keto diet for those readers who are middle aged is that it directly attacks every aspect of metabolic syndrome. If you think you might have metabolic syndrome or your doctor has told you that you have metabolic syndrome, going on a keto diet is the best thing that you can do for yourself. In fact, the keto diet will directly cure or eliminate metabolic syndrome provided that you carefully follow the diet and stick to it over the long-term.

Myths About the Keto Diet

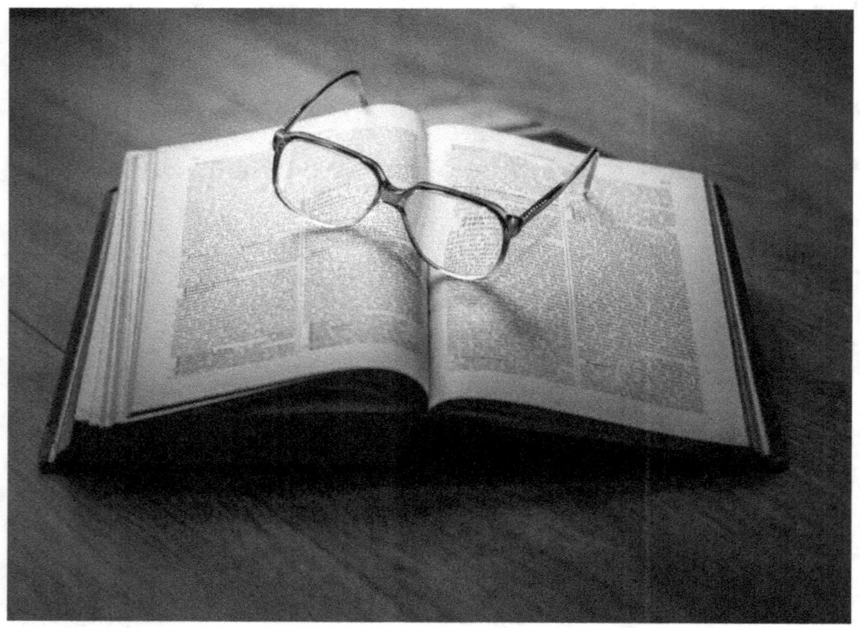

Unfortunately, the internet is swirling with myths about the keto diet. It's important to understand what these myths are, because you are likely to encounter them on different websites, many of which are considered authoritative on health issues.

We have already discussed the main myth that is promoted, and that is the myth that following a keto diet is going to cause "acidosis" or high levels of acid in the blood. Unfortunately, this myth is often promoted by nutritionists and medical professionals. They should know better, but the fact is they are threatened by the existence of the keto diet and the benefits it has. As a result, they promote this myth in order to try and discredit the diet. It's not clear if they do so as a result of pure ignorance or if they are actually lying about the diet. Many doctors – and supposed nutrition experts, many of whom are highly educated and 'certified' – may refused to look at information that contradicts their closely held beliefs about diet and nutrition. In fact, this is a common phenomenon in the sciences. When there are certain ideas that are considered to be "true facts" in science, those who have been brainwashed by these ideas, often for decades, find it impossible to give them up. They will create a mental blind spot that ignores evidence that is contradictory to what they believe. As a result, they will either use kneejerk dismissiveness when confronted with new evidence, or they will simply refuse to even examine it, discuss it, or hear about it.

One of the most amusing things when it comes to the keto diet, is you can read accounts of doctors who attend diabetes conferences where they are fed the kinds of foods that can lead to the development of diabetes. That is, they are given meals that contain a lot of carbohydrates including sugary fruits like bananas.

Ironically, if you develop diabetes the odds are that you are going to be sent to a counseling session with a "nutrition expert" who is going to advise you to eat a diet that is low in fact and high in carbohydrates. You might stop and think for a moment how absurd this is – that the medical establishment would advise people who have a disease related to carbohydrate consumption to eat more carbohydrates. But this is a basic fact about the world we live in and the way that the medical establishment is operating.

Unfortunately, the sad truth when it comes to the scientific enterprise and these kinds of tightly held beliefs is that the people holding them need to retire and move on before the establishment comes around fully to the new viewpoint. This is called a paradigm shift, and when it comes to fat and carbohydrate consumption, the medical establishment is going to have to undergo a paradigm shift. The views and beliefs that developed as a result of the theories promoted by Ancel Keyes are very well ingrained in the medical establishment even today.

In fact, you see many medical scientists and nutritionists actively fighting against the concept of a ketogenic diet, and against the consumption of animal fat. They either ignore or dismiss research showing the diet works or that saturated fat is not harmful.

This brings us to another myth associated with the keto diet, which is that it does not produce long term weight loss. Many will claim that the keto diet will lead to weight loss for awhile, but that over time people will gain the weight back. The fact is there are no studies that show this. People who quit the diet are going to gain the weight back, but the fact is that many people are able to stick to the keto diet over the long term. This is a personal commitment that you have to make for yourself. The recent development of "cyclic" keto, where you can take some time off to eat carbohydrates, is helping people stay on the keto diet long-term, by letting them satisfy their cravings. Other people don't have cravings for carbohydrate-based foods and don't need to do this. But keep in mind that after you have reached your weight loss goals, having occasional days where you consume carbohydrate-based foods works out fine, and it's not going to cause you to regain all of your weight.

Some of the myths that surround the keto diet come from absolute ignorance about it. One of the myths that is promoted is the idea that the diet is a high protein diet. In fact, nothing could be further from the truth. This myth in part comes from the Atkins diet, which does allow more protein consumption than a keto diet. However, the keto diet is a moderate protein diet, it is not a high protein diet. Anyone that makes the assertion that the keto diet is a high protein diet is not someone who has bothered to actually research the diet to find out what it involves.

Another myth about the keto diet that is making its way around is that it actually increases the risk of developing type 2 diabetes. Since type 2 diabetes is a disease that is associated with sugar intake, this myth is completely absurd to begin with! However, we don't need to just dismiss the claim. Multiple studies have actually shown that carbohydrate restriction helps prevent type 2 diabetes and it also helps manage diabetes for those who already have it, by helping to control blood sugar levels. Some studies even show that following a low-carb or ketogenic diet can reverse type 2 diabetes in 60% or more of patients.

Some also claim that the keto diet is not suitable for athletes. In fact, this is false. In the early stages of the diet, some people are going to have trouble adjusting, but these problems pass with time. During the initial phase athletes may find that their performance suffers, but they are also going to find – provided that they stick through the diet during the transition phase – that over time the diet is extremely beneficial. Many famous athletes are actually using the keto diet to help promote and maintain a better body composition (less fat and more muscle) such as NBA star Lebron James. The keto diet will help reduce the amount of body fat, and it also helps athletes improve recovery after hard workouts and training, according to several studies. The keto diet has even been found to help endurance athletes like marathon runners even though the long-term myth about that type of exercise is that you need to "carb load". Some studies have even shown that in head-to-head competitions, athletes following a low carb diet do better than those that are following a high carb diet.

Some medical professionals are going around promoting another myth, which is that the keto diet is bad for you because of low fiber intake. The reality is that the keto diet isn't a low fiber diet. There are other sources of dietary fiber than bread or pasta, and "whole grains". In fact, you are encouraged to eat a lot of green vegetables and avocados on a keto diet, and these foods contain plenty of fiber. In fact, avocados rank near the top if not at the top when it comes to dietary fiber content. If you are properly following the keto diet, which means eating plenty of vegetables, you are not going to have a problem with low fiber intake.

Another myth promoted by ignorant doctors and nutritionists is that the keto diet will cause gallbladder problems. It turns out that contrary to common belief, diets high in fat actually improve the health of the gallbladder. The increased production of bile can help clear out smaller gallstones, leading to better long-term health of the gall bladder. Other studies show that diets that are high in fat reduce the formation of gallstones in the future. It appears that the combination of fat and sugar is the biggest risk factor in the development of gallstones and gallbladder problems, but not the consumption of high fat alone.

Some medical professionals are going around promoting the idea that a keto diet can actually shorten your lifespan. This claim is based on an article that was published in the prestigious medical journal the Lancet, which was also popularized in the newspaper USA Today. However, something that is being left out of the discussions that came out of this article was that the people studied were not following the keto diet. In fact, the low carb group used in the study got 37% of their daily calories from carbohydrates. While that is lower than what people following a standard American diet consume (over 50%, typically up to 60%), a carbohydrate intake of 37% does not even count as low carb. The keto diet is very strict when it comes to carbohydrates, and on keto you are probably going to be eating 5% of your calories from carbs, 10% at the most. So, this study does not even apply.

Moreover, multiple studies have actually shown that low carb diets actually reduce the risk of death from multiple causes for most people. We know that being overweight and obese raises the risk of developing multiple diseases that can be fatal, so avoiding becoming overweight or obese, or reversing these conditions, is obviously going to massively benefit your health, not cause problems with it.

The final myth that we are going to examine is the claim that people lose weight on keto because they are eating fewer calories, but they aren't aware of it. Now in some cases people might eat fewer calories. However, the keto diet does not cause weight loss because you are eating fewer calories. The weight loss that people experience on keto is due to the reduction in the levels of insulin in their body, and the increased amount of time that glucagon levels are elevated. Remember how it works – insulin drives stored fat; glucagon burns stored fat. It's really that simple. That is the root cause of weight loss on keto. It is not something that is based on calorie or portion size restriction, at all.

Keto Weight loss Success

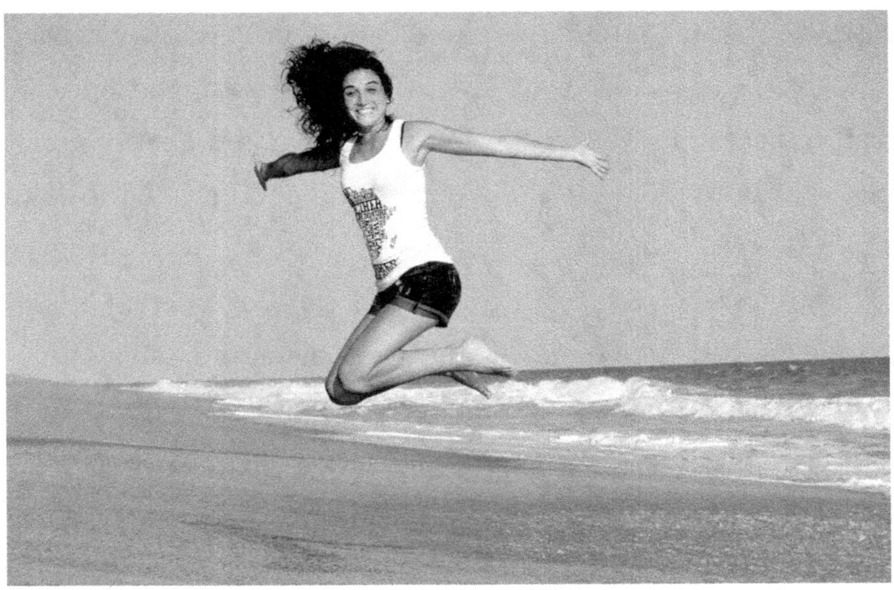

The keto diet has many advantages. In fact, calling it a diet is a misnomer, we should be referring to the keto diet as a lifestyle. A diet involves restricting calories. People on diets are hungry all the time because they are trying to lose weight by not getting the amounts of food that their bodies need in order to function properly. Even people who are not dieting, but who are eating a standard American diet, get really hungry between meals because that is how carbohydrates roll, as we discussed earlier. You burn them off quickly or they are stored as fat, and a couple of hours later your body is dying for food again.

Not so with the keto diet. As we discussed earlier the keto diet provides a steady source of energy and there are not the kinds of fluctuations that you are going to experience with "normal" eating patterns. Second, the keto diet doesn't' restrict calories or portion sizes at all. If you are properly following the keto diet, you eat until you don't want to eat anymore. That ensures that your body will have enough energy to get through the day, and certainly to the next meal.

People on the keto diet don't get hungry in between meals, or at the worst they might have moderate hunger. This fact makes the keto diet more sustainable. One of the reasons that people give up typical diets is that the hunger they experience, together with feelings of being weak and irritable that often come with falling blood sugar spikes, often lead them to give up their diets.

Studies have shown that it's possible to stick with a keto diet long term, and those that do experience sustained weight loss. Moreover, the amount of weight loss that people following a keto diet far outpaces that obtained with other diets. Some studies have looked at people that have followed the keto diet for 2 years or longer. Unfortunately, this isn't that easy to do because the keto diet has not been that popular for very long, it's really only gained significant traction over the past 2-3 years. Nonetheless, these studies have found that those who are able to stick to the diet for 2 years or longer maintain long-term weight loss.

Other studies that are not specifically geared toward the keto diet but that examine low carb diets in general, have found that low carb diets are better for weight loss than other types of dieting. In particular, they lead to more initial weight loss, and after periods of one year or more, people following a low carb diet are more likely to keep the weight off as compared to people who try other types of diets that involve calorie and portion restrictions. Many studies have reported that 75% of low carb dieters are able to lose 10 pounds or more and 33% of dieters are able to lose 30 pounds or more.

Browsing the internet, it's easy to find personal testimonials about the benefits of weight loss from the keto diet. Often, this is even true among those over the age of 50. Consider Suzanne Ryan, who wrote Simply Keto. She used the keto diet in her own situation when she weighed 289 pounds. She's tall for a woman at 5 feet 11 inches, but 289 pounds at that height is quite obese. After sticking to the keto diet Suzanne was able to drop 120 pounds. You can find before and after pictures of Suzanne online that are quite spectacular.

You may think that is an exception, but in fact that is the rule for people that stick to the keto diet. Caitlin Graham managed to lose 50 pounds over a short time period. In fact, she was able to drop the weight in a mere four months of time. So that's weight loss averaging 25 pounds a month. How would you feel losing 25 pounds a month? The thing about the keto diet is that you never feel hungry, even when having weight loss of that magnitude. In fact, my bet is that she felt more energetic than ever while losing all that weight. If you search on the internet you can also find her before and after photos.

Chapter 3: Foods to Eat on Keto

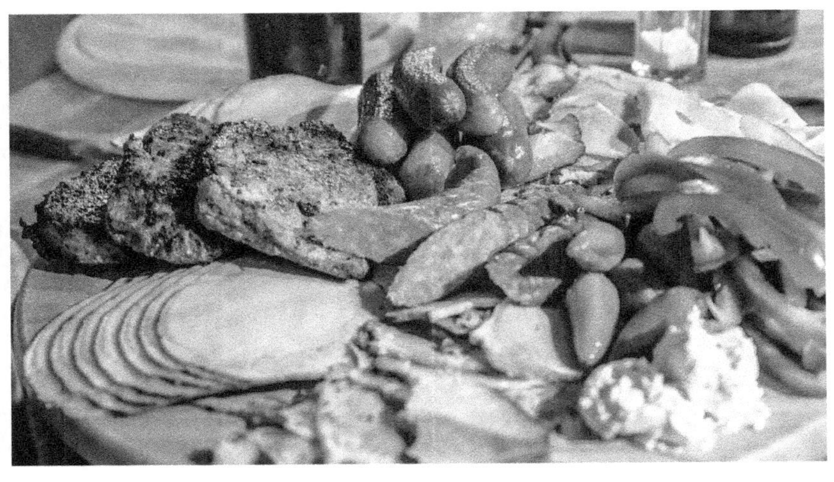

When you are starting on the keto diet, the first thing you need to do is to determine what foods you can eat on keto and what foods to avoid. The keto diet is not about controlling calories or portion sizes at all. So you can stop worry about that and you should never try to control the amount you eat when following the keto diet – simply eat the amount of food that satisfies you at each meal, and then don't eat again until your body tells you that you need to eat. One of the things that often happens on the keto diet is that people will find that they don't need to eat as often as they used to. But don't worry if that happens to you or not, that really isn't the important issue. The important factor with keto, or we should say the most important factor, is reducing your consumption of carbohydrates. In fact, at least in the beginning you want to get them down to a bare minimum of 5% of your total calories. After you have been on the diet for awhile and lost a significant amount of weight, you may be able to increase your consumption of carbohydrates a bit, but you should never go back to the standard way of eating if you want to continue to enjoy the benefits of keto over the long term.

In this chapter we are going to discuss the foods that you can eat and the foods that should be avoided while following the ketogenic diet.

What foods you can eat on keto

A ketogenic diet can be summarized as high fat, moderate protein, and low carbohydrate. Some people may argue over the exact amounts of each of these general food types that you can eat, but the details are less important than following some general rules.

Let's start with fat. This is actually a difficult one for some people because we have been brainwashed, many of us from day one, into thinking that fat is bad for you. The nutritional establishment is in a state of perpetual confusion, and so they have come to allow the consumption of some fats, at least temporarily. But you need to stop paying attention to the constant stream of health news that infuses both the internet and the mainstream media and news, and simply follow a few basic rules when it comes to fat.

The first thing that we need to clear up is trans-fat. Of all the fats that exist in the dietary world, trans-fat is the only type of fat that needs to be avoided. However, there needs to be some clarification on this issue. The reason is that trans-fat actually exists in natural and unnatural (or artificial) forms. Naturally occurring trans-fat is fine. It is found in beef products in relatively small amounts. Make sure that you remember this – naturally occurring trans-fats are not dangerous and they will only be consumed in small amounts anyway. A common source of naturally occurring trans-fats is in ground beef.

Artificial trans-fats are not good to consume. Of course, we are talking about consuming them on a regular basis. Consuming artificial trans-fats one time or now and then is not going to have any impact on your body. So, there is no reason to be neurotic about eating something that has trans-fats in it. That said, when consumed on a regular basis they can be a problem. Studies have shown that regular consumption of trans-fats wrecks havoc on your system. In particular, it does the exact opposite of what you want to happen to your blood lipids. Artificial trans-fats will raise your triglycerides, raise your bad or LDL cholesterol, and lower your good or HDL cholesterol all at the same time. By themselves, it appears they can cause heart disease.

Trans-fats were used for many decades in cooking, because they held up well with a long-shelf life. As a result, they were used in many processed foods, particularly those that were packaged and sold in grocery stores. Many restaurants routinely used them in cooking deep fried foods.

The good news about this is that the FDA has banned the use of trans-fats. Food companies were given a time period over which they could transition to using other types of oils in their products, but by the end of this year trans-fats (again we are talking about the harmful, artificial variety) will probably be gone from most or all food products.

Fats You Can Eat on Keto

Beyond trans-fats, you can eat any kind of fat on the keto diet. While you may want to get adequate or good levels of certain kinds of fats like the omega-3 fat found in fish, there are no rules about what kind of fats you should eat on keto. You can eat whatever fats and fatty foods satisfy your pallet. However, many people find that getting enough fat is a bit of a challenge when starting out. So, let's review some food items that you can consume while on the keto diet that can help you maintain a high level of fat intake.

- Bacon: Bacon can add to your fat intake in two ways. Of course, eating bacon for breakfast or as a part of other meals will increase your fat intake, especially if you don't cook it so that it's totally crisped. It can also do so by using the left-over bacon fat. A good way to incorporate bacon into a keto diet is by frying in in a pan, so that you can use the leftover grease. Then cook other foods in the bacon grease. A good thing that you can do is use bacon grease to cook spinach and other greens in. That way you are adding a lot of fat to what is otherwise a nonfat food.

- Avocados: Eating avocados frequently and even on a daily basis is good for many reasons, not the least of which is that they are a high fat food. One cup of chopped avocado contains 21 grams of fat. Adding a cup of avocado to your daily diet will go a long way toward helping you meet your needs for avocado in your diet. While avocados have a distinct flavor, it's somewhat bland as well and so mixes with many other foods and spices quite effectively, so that you can avoid getting tired of eating avocado by trying varied preparations. You can also easily add avocado to salads.

- Don't remove skin from poultry. Because of the many decades long brainwashing that the public has suffered through, many of use feel a need to eat skinless poultry. If you enjoy skinless poultry it can certainly be included in a keto diet, however you shouldn't be afraid of consuming poultry with the skin on either. In fact, you should try doing it more often. Chicken skin not only contains needed fat but it may be nutritious in surprising ways. It's well known that the advice from your grandmother to consume chicken soup for colds and flu is not a myth, and it appears that it's the chicken fat that helps. Also consider eating higher fat varieties of poultry like duck breasts.

- Don't remove fat from steaks. This is another ritual that stems from the brainwashing against fat that we've suffered through over the past several decades. We can imagine how insane our ancestors would think we were for cutting fat off a piece of meat, often to just throw away. Fat on meat would have been valued for its calorie content in ages past. And it should be now. If you want your meals to be more satisfying and longer lasting, then you should consume all the fat that is on a piece of meat. It will actually help you lose weight, rather than gain weight.

- Add butter or cream to your coffee. You can use butter and cream in your coffee to get some more fat. If you opt for using cream, use heavy cream. Don't use half-and-half, and don't use milk. Use heavy cream to taste. Keep in mind that heavy cream does contain trace carbohydrates. For those that like the taste, you can use butter in your coffee instead.

- Snack on nuts and seeds. Studies show that eating nuts and seeds significantly reduces the risk of heart disease and cancer. One reason for this is that they contain monounsaturated fats which have been shown to reduce inflammation. Nuts have varying levels of fat, but generally speaking nuts are considered a high-fat food. However, be sure to limit your intake of nuts. This is one food item that can put you at risk of overeating, and remember that they also contain some carbohydrates. In particular watch out for cashews and peanuts.

- Use butter and cheese in cooking. You should try and use lots of butter in your cooking to add some extra fat. You can also make cheese sauces, or mixtures of cheese and heavy cream to make good sauces that you can include with your meals to add more fat.

- Coconut cream. You probably want to avoid eating coconut or drinking coconut milk in large quantities because there is some carbohydrate content, however you can use coconut cream to get some more fat in your diet if you like the taste.

- Fat bombs: Snack on fat bombs to get more fat into your daily diet. You can find recipes for fat bombs online, but even some packaged food companies are selling fat bombs in stores. Just be aware of any carbohydrate content if you buy fat bombs premade. Even slimfast is selling fat bombs.

- Eat fatty fish – including the skin. Fatty fish is an excellent source of fat. In addition to simply adding more fat to the diet, fatty fish will provide you with omega-3 fats that are proven to lower triglycerides and help reduce the risk of heart attack and stroke. Many people avoid eating fish skin which is a mistake, it contains even more fat. The best fish to include in your diet are salmon, sardines, mackerel, anchovies, trout, and arctic char.

- Top foods with olive oil and avocado oil. You can always top off veggies or even meats with more oils that will help the flavor besides giving you more fat in your diet. After you've cooked a steak or piece of chicken, consider drizzling it with olive oil.

- Snack on cheese. When you buy cheese after adopting a keto diet, always get the full fat varieties. You can use cheese as an excellent snack when you feel like eating something in between meals. You can also add a few chunks of cheese to any meal, either as part of the meal or served on the side. Try higher fat varieties of cheese as well like brie. Cheese will help you feel satisfied, help you get more of your calories from fat, and makes a great snack.

Meats to Eat on Keto

Virtually any kind of meat can be consumed on the keto diet. If you are eating a low-fat type of meat like skinless chicken breasts or cod fish, cook it in butter or olive oil and consider topping it off with high fat sauces that include butter, cream, or olive oil.

Meats to include on keto include (but are not limited to):

- Steak of all types. Fattier cuts like rib eye and NY Strip steak are preferred.
- Ground beef, get higher fat varieties. You should eat 80/20 or 73%.
- Other cuts of beef, such as roast beef and prime rib. Note that grass fed beef is the best, but it's not required by any means.
- Equivalent cuts of bison are also good.
- Chicken, eat with skin on or top with fat containing sauces. Cook with lots of fat like added butter.
- Duck
- Turkey, including turkey skin.
- All pork products, when considering unprocessed meat.
- Sausage is ok. However, check the carbohydrate content. Some sausage might contain more carbohydrates than you think, and it needs to be counted. Don't eat low fat sausage.
- Fatty fish —as mentioned above eat salmon, mackerel, sardines, arctic char, trout, anchovies. Any fatty fish is acceptable. Don't eat breaded fish, however.

Now let's talk about processed meats. The notion that processed meats like salami are inherently dangerous is exaggerated. Should you eat them in large quantities? Probably not. But as an occasional part of your diet hot dogs, salami, pepperoni, ham, and other products are perfectly fine. These products often have the advantage of having high fat content. The only thing to really worry about when consuming these foods is that they sometimes contain carbohydrates. If you are eating hot dogs, for example, you might want to check the carb content before eating a large number of them. The amount of carbs may vary by manufacturer.

As far as worrying about nitrates, keep in mind that nitrates are naturally created when you eat food anyway. That's right, you actually make nitrates in your saliva. Also, there is a bit of a scam going on, many meats are sold as "uncured", when in fact they are cured using celery salt. In the end, the distinction on a chemical level is that there is no distinction. Also, the evidence that consuming nitrates and nitrites causes cancer isn't as solid as it's made out to be. Again, should you consume salami with every meal? Probably not – but snacking on it now and then is probably not only perfectly fine, it will also probably help you meet your goals with the keto diet.

Fruits

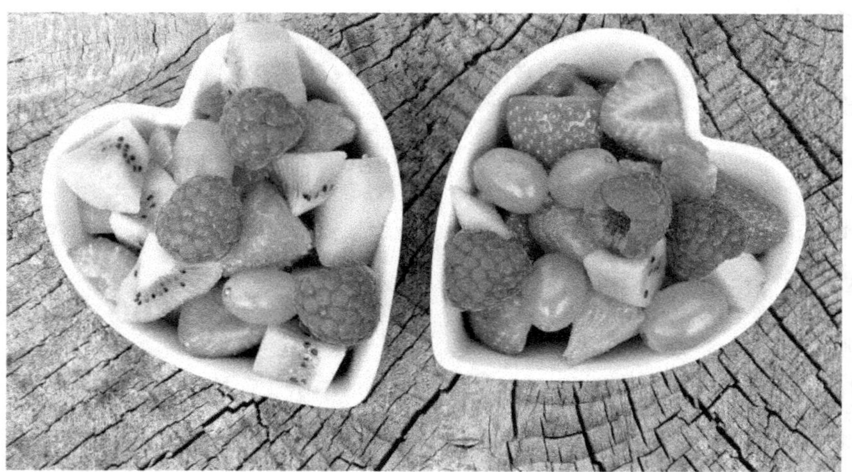

Fruit consumption needs to be strictly limited on the keto diet. This is because fruit is essentially sugar water. Of course, it's nutritious because it also contains lots of vitamins and minerals, however you are going to be able to get those vitamins and minerals from other sources. There are some fruits that you can consume, but the list is small. This is a hard one for some people to get past, because we have also been trained to believe that fruit consumption is an essential part of a healthy diet, and we've been led to believe that if we aren't getting several servings of fruit every day our health may be in danger. Frankly these notions are questionable, but there are some fruits that you can eat. We are going to list them here:

- Avocados: You can certainly eat avocados on a daily basis. Not only do they have lots of fat and dietary fiber which is going to really help your efforts on the keto diet overall, avocados are also packed with lots of vitamins and minerals.

- Olives: when you say fruit, olives are probably not the first thing that comes to mind. But olives are a fruit and you can get a serving of fruit by eating a handful of olives. You also get the side benefit that they contain healthy olive oil.

- Tomatoes: You can eat tomatoes in moderation. They make a great garnish in many dishes and you can add them to salads.

- Strawberries: Now we get into the realm of berries. You can eat strawberries, but do so in moderation. If you are consuming a lot of strawberries and find that you are not losing weight, consider cutting back or eliminating them.

- Blueberries: Ditto for blueberries. A healthy food packed with a lot of vitamins, minerals, and phytonutrients that your body needs, but consume in moderation.

- Blackberries: Blackberries have less sugar content that strawberries or blueberries.

- Raspberries: Believe it or not, raspberries have less sugar content than strawberries and blueberries as well, so you can eat them. All berries should be consumed in moderation, this is not a green light to eat as many as you feel like.

That is a good listing of a few fruits that you can continue consuming while on the keto diet, to satisfy your "requirements" for fruit consumption while avoiding the varieties that contain significant amounts of sugar (which is nearly all of them).

Vegetables

Contrary to myth, the keto diet is rich in vegetables. You are encouraged to eat lots of veggies with every meal. Primarily, you are going to want to eat leafy green vegetables. You can stir fry them or eat salads. Thinking in terms of a meat and salad diet is a great way to think of keto. Some vegetables that you can eat include:

- Arugula
- Celery
- Cauliflower
- Broccoli
- Spinach
- Mustard greens
- Turnip greens
- Cabbage
- Onions
- Leeks

- Asparagus

- Green beans

- Radishes

- Romaine lettuce

The list of vegetables is actually quite long, you are probably
going to want to look at the list of foods that you can't eat when
it comes to vegetables.

Foods to Avoid on Keto

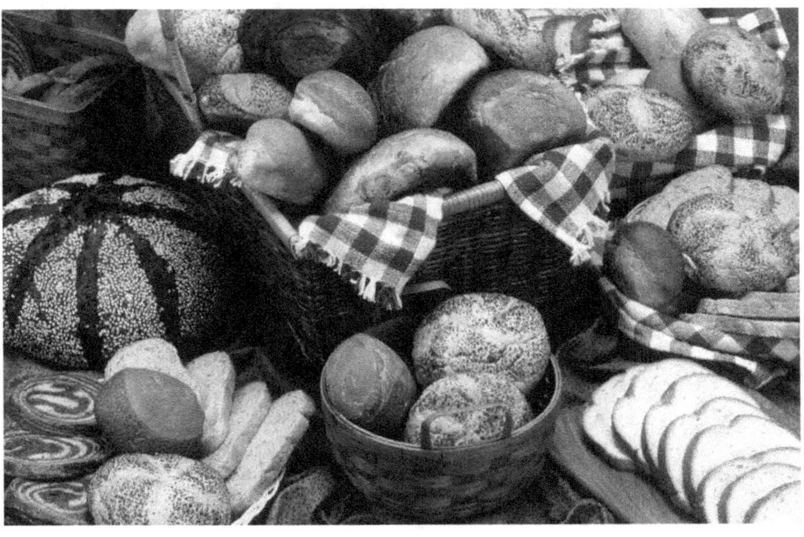

The list of foods to avoid on keto is actually based on a simple
principle, simply avoid carbohydrate-based foods. You know
what they are, just stop eating them. If you are starting keto it's
a good idea to go through your pantry and kitchen and either
throw out or giveaway any carbohydrate-based foods that are

taking up space. You want to avoid the temptation, and you are better off donating them to a food bank rather than keeping them around and possibly eating them in a moment of desperation.

Here is a listing of foods that you should avoid while following the keto diet:

- White rice
- Brown rice
- Quinoa
- Corn
- Blue corn
- Bread (all types)
- Oats
- Barley
- Buckwheat
- All cereals
- Hot cereals (just to be sure)
- Potatoes
- Sweet potatoes
- Couscous
- Pasta of all types
- Ice cream (unless you have a low sugar variety)
- Honey

- Molasses
- Sugar of all forms
- Salad dressings containing sugar except in very limited amounts (1 gm per serving)
- Soda
- Fruit juice
- All fruits containing sugar (give them away)
- Candy
- Beer
- Yogurt that contains sugar or fruit
- Milk
- Ketchup and any sugar containing condiments

Alcohol

The topic of alcohol deserves special mention. You don't need to give up alcohol on a keto diet, however there needs to be some care applied when consuming alcohol. First off, beer should be avoided while following a keto diet. If you are going to consume beer, it has to be on an infrequent basis, once a month at the most. Instead of trying to maintain your beer consumption you are better off getting off it entirely and drinking something else if you must continue consuming alcohol. You can consume dry wines. This includes red wines like merlot, zinfandel, and cabernet sauvignon.

Sugary wines should be avoided. Also avoid mixed drinks that contain any sugar or syrups. You can drink hard liquor, either plain or mixed with plain soda, perhaps with a lime. Avoid mixed drinks like margaritas, pina coladas, and white Russians, to name just a few. Many mixed drinks have sugar and syrups in them. Also avoid tonic water which contains sugar. You can drink pure brandy, which has zero carbohydrates. Avoid so-called bum or cheap wines, these have high sugar content.

Keto on a Budget

One of the myths that accompanies the keto diet is that it has to be expensive. Certainly, it can be expensive, if you are eating salmon and rib eye steaks at every meal. However, while those are good keto foods, you don't have to eat them to do well on keto.

In fact, for many meals you can use low cost lunch meat to get your protein. In that case, just be sure to add lots of fat to your meals because lunch meat is usually pretty low fat. You can make lunch meat plates to take to work for lunch. Just remember to skip the bread. A lunch meat plate can include the lunch meat of your choice, a cup of cubed avocado, some cheese, and a salad. You can drizzle the meat with olive oil or dip in full fat mayo to get some flavor.

Other foods that can be good on a keto diet on a budget include canned sardines, Vienna sausages (yes – great keto food with high fat and moderate protein), eggs, and hot dogs (again watch the carbs). You can eat hot dogs with mustard or full fat mayo. Remember of course that you can't eat the bun when consuming hot dogs, and don't eat corn dogs.

Hamburger is also good. You can stir fry it in a pan or cook patties topped off with cheese. Many people like hamburgers where you use romaine lettuce for the bun, but fair warning that can be a little bit messy. Just avoid using ketchup, which is high in sugar.

Canned tuna can also be included on a low budget keto diet. These days, it's possible to get tuna that is packed in olive oil. Don't drain the olive oil and throw it out – that is good calories from fat that you need. You can make tuna salads as another way to include low cost proteins in your keto diet on a budget.

Consider snacking on celery using high fat dips that are low in carbs. Always read your labels so that you can be sure that you are not getting too many carbohydrates in your diet. Sometimes sauces and dips have hidden carbohydrates that can add up. You can also make your celery more satisfying by filling it with full fat cream cheese, that adds both fat and calories that your body needs.

Your friends and coworkers might be laughing at you when you are eating hot dogs without a bun, but they aren't going to be the ones laughing when you lose a whole bunch of weight as a result.

Chapter 4: Dealing with Keto Problems

When starting a keto diet, you may experience some problems that arise when your body is weaning itself from sugar and adjusting to getting its energy from other sources. In this chapter we are going to go over the top problems that people get when starting a keto diet and how to overcome them. As we will see often these problems arise from not having the proper diet, and so the problems are not really from the keto diet itself.

Keto Flu

Many people experience a phenomenon that has come to be called the "keto flu" during the first week or two of the diet. This experience is typically accompanied by fatigue, irritability, insomnia, and headaches. Some people even experience dizziness and nausea. Keto flu is not an imaginary phenomenon, and many people experience it and they attribute it to the keto diet itself. As a result, some people will use this as an excuse to quit the keto diet.

The main cause of the keto diet is carbohydrate deprivation. In short, your body has been addicted to carbohydrates over a lifetime, and breaking it cold turkey is difficult. This is the main source of the fatigue that you experience while suffering from the keto flu. The good news is that over time, your body will adjust. And the time frames that are involved are not that long. For many people the keto flu will pass in a matter of days. Certainly – assuming that you don't mess yourself up by giving into the temptation to cheat – you should be past the keto flu by the second week of the diet.

Another problem that can lead to the keto flu or make it worse is an electrolyte imbalance. Switching to the keto diet can be a big change as are as our electrolyte consumption. You can develop deficiencies in salt, calcium, magnesium, and potassium. Yes, you heard that right – when you switch to a keto diet you can actually develop a deficiency in salt. That is another one of those things that can be hard to believe because we've been told over and over again for decades that salt is bad for you and that everyone should be cutting back on salt.

However, sodium levels can drop in the body when you make the switch to keto, and this can create problems. Part of the reason that this can happen is that insulin is involved in keeping the kidneys regulating mineral balances in the body. When you go on keto your body is going to have to readjust for this and this can take a few days. Also, remember that on keto you are going to be burning off glycogen in your liver. Remember that each molecule of glycogen is linked to four molecules of water. So, when your body breaks down glycogen into individual glucose molecules, the water is going to be released as well.

And what happens to that water? You urinate it out. In fact, in the first week or two on the keto diet many people find that they are urinating a lot more than normal. This is not something to be worried about in and of itself, but the problem is that when you are urinating a lot, you are losing a lot of important minerals from your body. This includes sodium, potassium, calcium, and magnesium.

As it is, many Americans are already magnesium deficient. If magnesium deficiency becomes serious enough, you can develop severe fatigue, have muscle cramps and even muscle weakness, and develop dizziness. Magnesium deficiency can be closely linked to keto flu.

Heart Palpitations

Heart palpitations are one symptom that some people develop when starting the keto diet. This symptom is closely related to the causes of keto flu. In particular, heart palpitations are related to sodium and magnesium deficiencies. So, one thing that you need to be considering when starting a keto diet is whether or not you are getting enough magnesium in your diet.

Muscle Cramps

Muscle cramps are a common complaint when starting keto. This is another problem that is directly related to electrolyte depletion. To keep your muscles functioning healthy, you need adequate levels of sodium, potassium, and magnesium.

Getting your electrolytes back on track

The first thing to do if you are experiencing these symptoms – and in fact anyone who is on the keto diet should be following this advice – is to look at and adjust your mineral intake. First let's have a look at sodium. Getting enough salt is going to be an issue with the keto diet, and although you might be a little bit hesitant because of all the things about salt that people have been telling you over the past several years, you need to increase your salt intake on keto. Insulin helps the body hold onto sodium and when your insulin levels are low all the time, as they are going to be on a keto diet, your body is not going to hold onto sodium as well as it used to be. That means that you need to consume more salt to make up for the difference.

The standard recommendation for salt intake is 2,400 mg per day. In fact, this is far too low on a keto diet. On keto, at a minimum you should be consuming 3,000 mg per day, and some people should be consuming up to 5,000 mg per day. But you shouldn't have to sit around and try measuring the salt that you are eating. Let your body be the guide. If your body needs salt, you will find that you are craving salt. A good rule to follow is to salt your food to taste. This is a simple way to help ensure that you are getting enough salt.

Everyone should salt their food on keto, but the amount of salt you use will depend on how much you personally need.

Now we come to magnesium. This is important for relieving heart palpitations and muscle cramps. It turns out that there are some good natural sources of magnesium, but you can also take supplements. Be aware that magnesium is a laxative in large doses. So, if you decide to take a supplement, try 250 mg per day and see how that works. If you are comfortable with it and it still doesn't relieve symptoms of muscle cramps and heart palpitations, then you can consider moving up to 500 mg a day.

But let's take a look at some good natural sources. The first one to consider is avocados. These have large amounts of magnesium and potassium, so you can eat an avocado a day and kill two birds with one stone.

You can also get a lot of magnesium from nuts. Generally, the consumption of nuts should be limited while on a keto diet, but you can eat a handful of nuts or seeds a day. It turns out that nuts of all varieties contain high levels of magnesium. A handful is not going to be enough to satisfy your entire daily needs, however, it will certainly contribute and combined with some avocado will get you a long way toward your goals.

You can also get magnesium from spinach. Try eating a cup of spinach a day in salads or stir fried. This will also help increase your potassium.

Now let's have a look at potassium. This important mineral is important for keeping up your muscle strength and also to avoid muscle cramps. Potassium depletion can contribute to many of the problems addressed already, including heart palpitations, muscle weakness, and muscle cramps. An adult should consume around 4,000-5,000 mg of potassium per day. You can get 1,000 mg of potassium in a whole avocado. Other good sources of potassium include beef, chicken, and fish. You can also get potassium by eating almonds or walnuts. In the unlikely event you need to supplement with potassium, try using salt substitute to add more of it to your food. However, if you eat the foods above getting enough potassium shouldn't be much of an issue.

To get calcium, you can start by adding some cheese to your diet, which is an excellent source of dietary calcium. In addition, you can eat foods like broccoli and spinach. If in doubt, consider supplementing. This is fine for women but men are not recommended to supplement because this can increase the risk of heart disease for men by encouraging more calcium to go into the arteries.

Constipation or Diarrhea

Another problem that people run into when starting the diet is digestive problems. First, let's address diarrhea. If you suffer from this issue when starting the keto diet, this is because your body is having difficulty handling the large amounts of fat that you may not be used to. The first thing to note in this case is that with time, the body will adjust, and get used to it and it will pass. However, you can help the adjustment period with a gradual transition. If you are having some difficulties dealing with the high amounts of fat, try starting out with lower amounts of fat and gradually increase the levels of fat in your diet. During the transition period, you can keep carbohydrate consumption lower and eat more protein. So, each day as you progress, you will cut back a little bit on protein and add more fat. The diarrhea problem should clear up in a week or so.

Constipation problems are actually more common on the keto diet. Usually, this is a result of not getting enough fiber, but it can also be caused by electrolyte imbalances. So, you are going to want to look at both factors. Remember that magnesium is a laxative so magnesium deficiency might be a contributing factor here. But in most cases, not getting enough fiber is the culprit. This happens because prior to going on a keto diet, people are getting most of their fiber from bread and pasta. When they suddenly cut out these foods, they are not adding other foods in to make up for the loss of fiber.

One thing to consider is to add an artificial fiber like Metamucil to your daily routine. You might do that on a temporary basis. Just make sure that whatever fiber supplement you use, it does not contain any added sugar.

You can also add high fiber keto foods to your diet to make up for the deficiency. Once again, avocados come to the rescue.

Avocados are a unique fruit in that almost all of the carbohydrates in an avocado are in the form of fiber. So, eating one avocado per day is going to go a long way toward making sure that you are getting enough fiber in your diet. Hopefully you have noticed a pattern here, avocados are the solution for almost any problem on a keto diet. So, you can knock out most of them all at once by starting to eat avocados on a daily basis. Be sure to add some salt.

Many nuts also contain respectable amounts of dietary fiber, so snacking on nuts is another way to make sure that you are getting enough fiber. You can also get decent amounts of fiber by eating plenty of salads or stir-fried greens, and by eating some broccoli. Consider also adding green beans to your diet.

Hydration

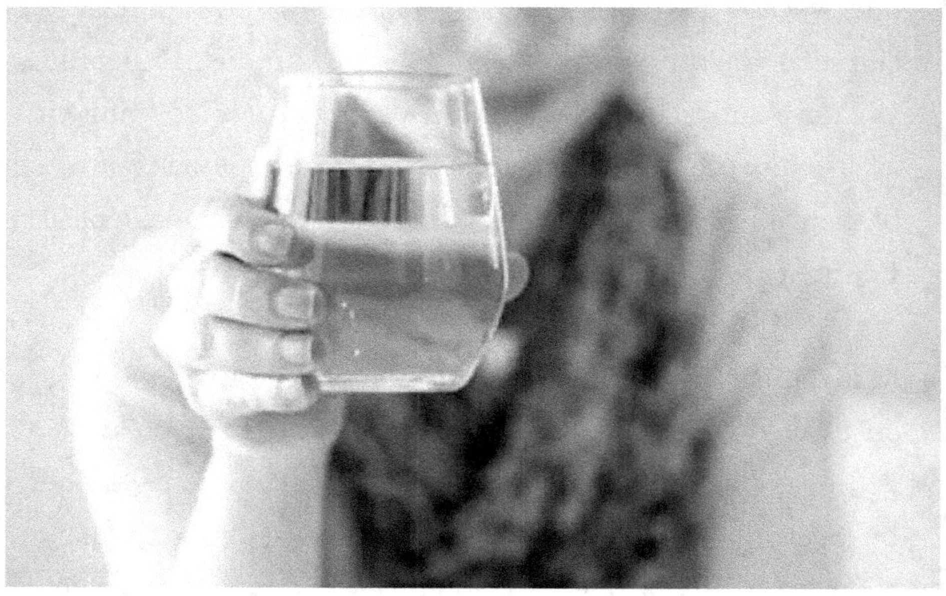

Another problem that happens when people start the keto diet is, they are not getting enough water. Remember that when you first start, your body is going to be getting rid of all the water that is stored in your liver with the glycogen. That means you are going to need to drink a lot of water to stay hydrated, since you might be urinating a lot more during the first couple of weeks of the diet. Pay special attention to getting enough water to keep everything in balance. Water can also help reduce any feelings of hunger, especially if you are incorporating fasting into your diet.

Chapter 5: How to Start Keto for Beginners

When starting the keto diet, there are a few rules that you should keep in mind to make sure that you are really doing a keto diet. In this chapter we will talk about the right ratios of macros and some other topics.

Macros

The macros that you consume on a diet are simply the percentage of fat, protein, and carbohydrates. The keto diet is considering a high fat, moderate protein, and low carbohydrate diet. We can start with the amount of carbohydrates, which is by far the most important part of the diet.

Carbohydrate consumption can be limited either by considering the amount, which is easier, or by considering the percentage of total calories consumed. In the latter case, the amount of carbohydrates should be limited to 5-10% of your total caloric intake. If you want to look at the total amount of carbohydrates consumed, you should eat 20 grams or less of carbohydrates per day. After you have met your weight loss goals, you may be able to increase the amount of carbohydrates consumed daily up to around 50 grams per day, and some people even do OK on 100 grams per day – after they have met their weight loss goals. At any point you can cut back again if you find that increasing the amount of carbohydrates causes problems.

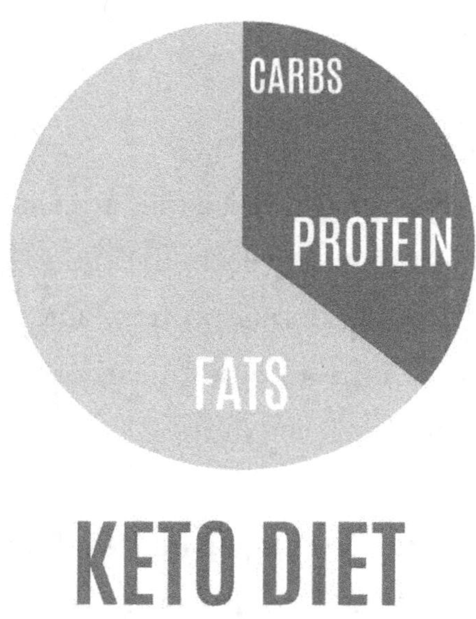

KETO DIET

When we are talking about consuming a given number of grams of carbohydrate, keep in mind that this is going to be net carbohydrates. So, for any food, take the total carbohydrates and subtract the number of grams of fiber that are contained in the food. That will give you the number of net carbohydrates.

Next, let's consider protein. Again, you can either focus on the percentage of calories or the number of grams that you eat. As a percentage of calories, you can aim for 15-20% of daily calories from protein. However, a good way to do it is to simply eat one gram of protein per pound of lean body mass. So, you will need to get an estimate of the amount of body fat you have. If you weigh 200 pounds and you are 40% body fat, then your lean body mass is 120 pounds. So, you can eat 120 grams of protein per day using this method.

So, we've hit two out of the three bases, the last thing to consider is fat, and your fat should range between 70-80% of total calories consumed.

Of course, to see if your diet is working, rather than doing these sorts of calculations you can track your ketones and blood sugar using a meter. If your ketones are between 1-3 mmol/L, then you are in good shape and should keep doing what you are doing.

Your First Week on Keto

The first week on keto is going to involve burning off your glycogen and making sure that you are not suffering from keto flu and other problems. We have given you the advice you need to deal with the first weeks problems effectively in the last chapter, so make sure that you are properly hydrated, and also that you are getting plenty of the minerals sodium, magnesium, potassium, and calcium, along with plenty of dietary fiber.

If you find yourself getting carb cravings, try eating something fatty to get rid of them. Coconut cream is good to have around for this purpose. Although it has negligible carb content, coconut cream has a bit of a sweet bite to it, and so a spoonful of it can help you eliminate or reduce cravings for carbohydrates. It's very high in fat so should actually help, rather than hinder, your weight loss efforts.

Fat Bombs to Conquer Hunger

We mentioned fat bombs earlier. You can search the internet to find recipes but now you can even buy them either online or in many stores. Fat bombs are a good snack to help you combat hunger during the early phases of keto. Just don't overdo it, you want to get out of the habit of snacking. But if you are not feeling satisfied don't be afraid to eat some delicious fat bombs. As we said earlier, if you buy fat bombs from the store make sure they are sugar free or very low in sugar.

Keto and Exercise

Keto can work very well with exercise, but for many people it is going to take some time for your body to adjust. For that reason, you might want to scale back your exercise efforts the first week or two on the diet if you are not feeling energetic.

This should pass with time, however, as the body learns to get its energy from fat sources.

Many experts advise taking it slow with exercise the first two weeks of the diet. You may not be quite sure how your body is going to respond with low blood sugar, but most people don't have problems. If you are used to exercising vigorously, try some light work outs until you are sure how your body will respond.

This advice applies primarily to aerobic exercise. Weight lifting can proceed normally without worrying too much. The best advice is to go with how you feel. If at any time during exercise you feel light headed or unusual, stop and eat a fat bomb or some other quick keto snack. However, this type of reaction is rarely reported. Most people who are starting keto find that the problem with exercise is usually that they are sluggish at first. This should pass after the first two weeks.

If you are sluggish with exercise, you might consider that this could be a problem that is related to electrolyte depletion. Make sure that you are getting enough sodium, potassium, and magnesium. If you are getting muscle cramps that are not normal for you when it comes to exercise, the problem can often be pinpointed to low levels of electrolytes.

You should avoid sports drinks when it comes to exercising, because many of them either contain sugar or artificial sweeteners. Small amounts of artificial sweeteners are OK on a keto diet, but consuming them in large amounts is discouraged. If you want to replenish electrolytes after exercise, consider drinking some bone broth. Many varieties of bone broth will contain some of the minerals that you need. You can also add a magnesium tablet if you are suffering from muscle cramps.

Chapter 6: Keto and Type 2 Diabetes

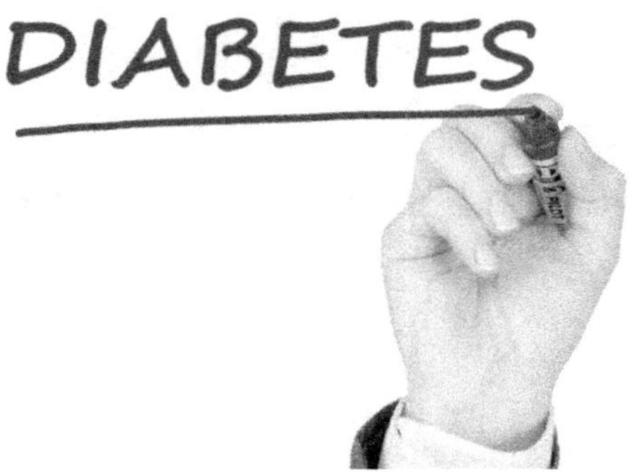

The keto diet may be one of the best things that has come along in some time for diabetes. Finally, rather than advising people who have problems metabolizing carbohydrates to eat more carbohydrates, we have a diet that can actually keep insulin levels low, reduce the need for insulin, and keep blood sugars under control. If you don't have diabetes but are at risk either because of a family history, being overweight, or because you already have pre-diabetes, a keto diet can help you prevent diabetes. If you already have diabetes, it's possible you can reverse it, although not everyone is able to do so. But at the very least, you will probably be able to mitigate it and reduce your dependence on medications.

If you have diabetes already, please consult with a doctor before adopting the keto diet. If your doctor is hostile about it you might consider finding a second opinion.

Some doctors might be put off by the keto diet, but the truth is you can think of the keto diet as a diet that is almost made for type 2 diabetes. My mother was diabetic and passed away before the keto diet was popular. Back in those days, she was always advised to eat low fat diets, and to consume large amounts of carbohydrates! Looking back on it just makes me angry to think about it, and I often wonder how she could have been helped by a keto diet.

Why is Keto good for diabetes?

The answer to this is quite simple. Diabetes can be said to be the sugar disease. It's a result of the body's inability to handle the digestion of sugar. What the ultimate cause is might vary from person to person, maybe it's due to the way your cells react to insulin. In fact, that is just details. The real cause can be traced to carbohydrate-based foods. Get rid of the carbohydrates, and you get rid of the diabetes. The earlier that you tackle this problem, the better off you are going to be. If you have been diagnosed as pre-diabetic but you are not yet on any medications like metformin, you are the best positioned person to reverse your illness before it becomes a problem. However, anyone who is diabetic might be able to do something about this problem by following a ketogenic diet. It may be possible to reduce and even eliminate medications.

Diabetics should also consider incorporating intermittent fasting into their lifestyle. This is an extra kick that can help you get the most out of following a ketogenic diet. See chapter 7 for details on this.

When you are eating high fat and low carb foods, you don't even need insulin. Following this type of diet will also help to reset the body. Insulin resistance can be reduced a great deal – by simply reducing insulin levels in the body. Second, by not eating carbohydrates you get at the root cause of type 2 diabetes. People who are pre-diabetic or diabetic are going to find that their fasting blood sugar drops by a lot. Furthermore, when you are eating a high-fat and low-carb diet, your blood sugars are never going to spike. This will help reduce the damage to the body that is often caused by diabetes.

Many people are going to find that moving to a low carb diet is going to dramatically improve the health status of anyone who is pre-diabetic or diabetic. Once you adopt this diet, the old ways of doing things are going to seem downright medieval. You are going to wonder why nutritionists are still running around recommending that diabetics eat lots of fruit (aka sugar), whole grains (aka sugar with fiber) and low-fat diets.

Preventing Type 2 Diabetes in the first place

If you are overweight or obese, but you don't have diabetes, make no mistake you are at elevated risk for developing it. Therefore, it's a good idea to consider strictly adhering to the keto diet. By getting those extra pounds off the body, you will massively decrease your risk of developing diabetes. Also, as mentioned in the last paragraph, you will have a lot less insulin circulating in the body if you are following a keto diet carefully. The less insulin you have circulating in your blood stream, the less insulin resistant your cells are going to become, putting your body in a healthier state that is further away from diabetes. Being overweight is in itself a symptom of insulin resistance.

Keto and Blood Sugar

The keto diet is proven to reduce fasting blood sugar levels in most people. You do have to give it time, the first week that you are on the keto diet, you might not notice much if any changes to your blood sugar. However, you are going to find that if you are able to stick to the diet for a few months that your fasting blood sugars are going to start dropping. Many people who have fasting blood sugars in the 120s or higher find that their fasting blood sugar will drop to 110 or below, even 100 or below, after a few months on the keto diet.

If you are already diagnosed as diabetic and you are also on medication, you will have to be careful about this. Some adjustment of your medication may be necessary, as you don't want to get in a situation where you might become hypoglycemic. For this reason, diabetics that are on medication including oral medications as well as using insulin injections may require medical supervision before using a keto diet plan.

Getting off Medications

Can you get off medications with the keto diet? Many people do. For one thing, the medications that people have to take on diabetes are designed for managing blood sugar. If you are not consuming carbohydrates in sufficient quantities, these medications can become irrelevant. However, the situation is going to vary from person to person. This is something that you are going to have to discuss with a physician, and careful monitoring may be necessary. Certainly, insulin injections can be reduced if not eliminated. Oral medications may possibly be reduced as well.

Type 1 Diabetes

We can't say whether or not a type 1 diabetic can follow a ketogenic diet, if or a loved one are interested in a ketogenic diet but type 1 diabetes is an issue, this is something that will have to be discussed with a physician and done under medical supervision. Generally, type 1 diabetics aren't considered suitable for a keto diet, but that is something you will have to decide with your doctor.

Chapter 7: Intermittent Fasting and Keto

Many people who are on the keto diet supercharge it by also following intermittent fasting. The word "Fasting" might strike fear and trepidation into the hearts of some, but in fact fasting in the way that most people do it is not any big deal at all. In fact, you are already doing intermittent fasting – you fast each night when you go to bed, assuming that you're not getting up in the middle of the night in order to eat. If you are that is a habit that you need to eliminate.

What is intermittent fasting?

First, lets recognize that the fasting state of the body is the same state that the body is in when following the ketogenic diet. That is, insulin levels are low and glucagon is active. If you have used up the stores of glycogen in your liver, you will be burning body fat when you are fasting.

Every time you go several hours without eating, you are basically fasting. So, fasting is nothing like starvation or anything crazy. It is simply going several hours without consuming any food. When you sleep overnight you are fasting. Many people skip breakfast, so they are already doing intermittent fasting. The simplest way to do intermittent fasting is to wait until lunch the next day in order to eat.

If you can avoid eating after 8 PM in the evening, this is a good step toward moving the body into intermittent fasting. Some fasting methods are more extreme than others, and some people even go a full 24 hours without eating. Whether or not you try something like that will depend on the state of your health.

The Effects of Fasting on the Body

Intermittent fasting has several benefits. If you are on a keto diet, you are already realizing many of them. When you are in a fasting state, your body is using the hormone glucagon in order to burn body fat for fuel. As a result, people who use intermittent fasting will find that they are able to lose weight, stabilize blood sugars, increase their mental clarity – and get many of the same benefits that you get while following the ketogenic diet. However, intermittent fasting also triggers an important process called autophagy.

Autophagy is a repair mechanism that the body uses to clear out the dead wood, so to speak. When autophagy is going on at a large level, your immune cells are eating up bad and old cellular components and old cells that no longer work. It's sort of like taking an old car in for a tune up. Autophagy literally means to eat yourself, and that is how it can be understood. Old cellular components are destroyed and replaced by new ones, which helps your body's cells function better. In addition, if the cells are too old and too far gone, they are destroyed altogether, so it is a process of renewal.

It is believed that autophagy can help the body stay young, and that this process may reduce the risk of contracting many of the chronic diseases that plague developed societies. So, you can reduce your risk for cancer, Alzheimer's, and other diseases that are associated with old age.

In order for autophagy to take place, your liver must have its glycogen stores depleted. This is a triggering mechanism for autophagy. This is one reason why fasting fits in tightly with the ketogenic diet. When you are on keto, your liver isn't going to have a huge supply of glycogen to burn off.

16/8 Intermittent Fasting

The question is how do you go about fasting? The answer is simple – you just avoid eating for a certain time period. You can drink plenty of water during fasting, and staying hydrated is highly recommended.

The first and most popular style of intermittent fasting is called 16/8. The idea behind this is simple. You eat all of the food you are going to consume over an eight-hour window. You can schedule this window at any time that works for you. The only thing that most people recommend is that you don't eat past 8 PM at night.

Other than that, there is nothing more to this method of fasting. It's very easy to follow and most people adapt to it rather easily. For many people, it will be hardly noticeable. You can take it further, by restricting your eating window even more. So, you could eat over a 7-hour, 6 hours, or even 4-hour time frame if you wanted. But, it's not necessary in order to realize the benefits. So, you can do what is best for you.

One Meal a Day

Some people take this to an extreme, and only eat one meal per day. They consume their entire days calories within one hour. Many people find this works for them and it helps them keep the pounds off. You can think of this as 23/1 fasting, so it's just an extreme version of what we described above.

Full Day Fasting

If you feel like you really need to reset your system, you can try fasting for a full 24-hour period. This might be advisable for diabetics or those who have cancer and want to incorporate a keto diet into their treatment plan. In either case, you should work under a doctor's supervision.

5/2 Fasting

This type of fasting incorporates two days of complete 24 hour fasting a week. So, if your two days are Tuesday and Thursday, on those days you won't consume anything except water.

Eat, Stop, Eat

This method of fasting seems to be carrying things to an extreme, but it involves only eating every other day. It's not clear that there are any additional benefits to making your fasting more intense if you are on the ketogenic diet, but if this is something that is of interest to you, search online for more information.

Integrating Intermittent Fasting with The Keto Diet

Integrating intermittent fasting with the keto diet is extremely easy. This is because your body is in the fasting state already. However, some people recommend using intermittent fasting to start the keto diet. In this case, they recommend that before you go on the keto diet, you fast for a complete 24-hour period. Then when your fast is over, you start the keto diet. I am not aware of any scientific studies that have been done looking at this approach, but it sounds like an interesting way to jump start the first week of the keto diet. Some cancer researchers that advocate for a keto diet also recommend an initiation period that involves fasting for at least 24 hours. That may be beneficial, but that is probably something you should discuss with your doctor.

Who should avoid fasting?

One question that can come up is who, if anyone, should avoid fasting. For starters, children and adolescents should not be allowed to fast. This can create an unhealthy relationship with food, and unlike the adult body, a growing body needs a constant supply of nutrients in order to be in optimal health. Young people can take up the keto diet, but fasting is probably inadvisable.

Second, women need to proceed with care. Certainly, women can do 16/8 fasting, but some of the more intense methods of fasting have proven to be problematic with some women. You should only do what you are comfortable with, and if you notice anything unusual such as missed periods, then you've gone too far in your fasting intensity and should scale it back.

Pregnant women or women who are breast feeding definitely should not use intermittent fasting.

Type 2 diabetics, for the most part, can probably use intermittent fasting and it will probably really help their condition. However, you should definitely speak to your doctor before trying this on your own. Remember that you might develop blood sugar issues like hypoglycemia, and so you might need to adjust your medication during or after fasting. This is definitely something that should be done under medical supervision if you are a type 2 diabetic.

Type 1 diabetics should avoid intermittent fasting altogether.

Intermittent Fasting and Other diets

One of the benefits of intermittent fasting is that it can be used with any diet. Therefore, while the keto diet works best with intermittent fasting, other diets work perfectly fine with it as well. They may not work as well because if you are eating a lot of carbs, you are going to be devoting a lot of the time fasting to clearing out your glycogen stores that get replenished every time that you consume large amounts of carbohydrates.

One thing to consider for those who are on the keto diet, is that if you find yourself occasionally cheating, or you are eating carbs on purpose now and then, you can use fasting to reset your body and get back on the keto diet. So, if you have a cheat day, consider fasting the following day. It doesn't have to be a complete fast but could be as simple as waiting until the evening to eat a single meal for that day. So, you would do a "one meal a day" just for the day following your cheat day.

Chapter 8: 21 Days Meal Plan

In this chapter we are going to include some suggestions for a 21 days meal plan. This will help you get started with the keto diet. It is certainly not a set of rules, you can eat anything you want on the keto diet as long as you aren't drawing from the banned food lists that we mentioned earlier.

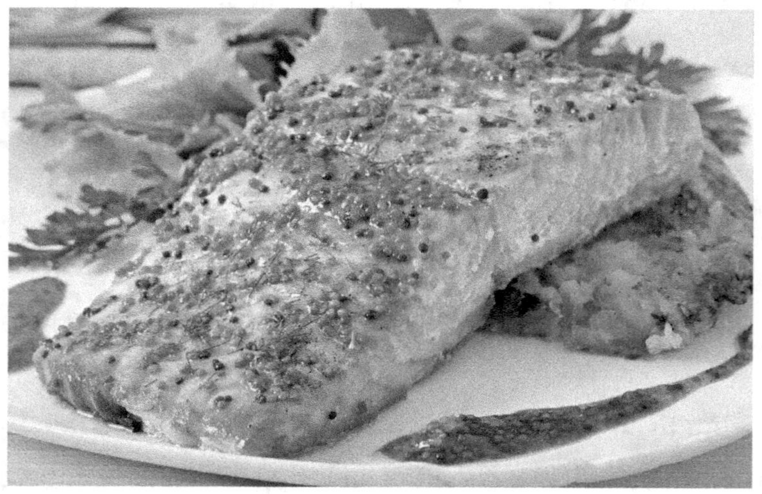

Week One

Sunday

Breakfast: Scrambled Eggs with 2 strips of bacon.

Lunch: Tuna Salad.

Dinner: Ribeye steak and green beans.

Monday

Breakfast: Avocado and smoked salmon.

Lunch: Roast beef lunch meet with mustard, diced and seasoned avocado, and cubed cheese.

Dinner: Grilled salmon and asparagus.

Tuesday

Breakfast: Sliced breakfast sausage with strawberries.

Lunch: Chicken Salad.

Dinner: Baked chicken thighs with parmesan cheese, spinach stir fried with mushrooms.

Wednesday

Breakfast: Cheese 3-egg omelet.

Lunch: Hamburger patty on a bed of greens.

Dinner: Chicken breasts in cream sauce with salad greens.

Thursday

Breakfast: Fried eggs and bacon.

Lunch: Cheese rollups, with deli meat of your choice, and tomato and arugula salad with low carb dressing.

Dinner: Lamb steaks with butter and rosemary, with mushroom, tomato, and spinach stir fry.

Friday

Breakfast: Smoked salmon and cream cheese.

Lunch: Spinach or arugula salad with avocado, slices of roast chicken, bacon slices, and goat cheese.

Dinner: Baked or broiled chicken wings with salad.

Saturday

Breakfast: Bullet coffee.

Lunch: Sardine salad.

Dinner: Baked trout with asparagus.

Week Two

Sunday

Breakfast: Ham and egg omelet.

Lunch: Smoked salmon and spinach plate.

Dinner: Baked Italian sausage with salad greens.

Monday

Breakfast: Bullet Coffee with smoked salmon.

Lunch: Sliced tomatoes, 3 olives, and can of tuna in olive oil.

Dinner: Pork chops with ¼ cup blueberries, and green beans.

Tuesday

Breakfast: Two over easy eggs with slice of ham or Canadian bacon in the middle with cheese.

Lunch: Classic tuna salad.

Dinner: Prime rib with asparagus.

Wednesday

Breakfast: 2 hard boiled eggs

Lunch: Cobb Salad with roast beef.

Dinner: Sliced sirloin steak stir fried with spinach and tomatoes in butter.

Thursday

Breakfast: Scotch eggs.

Lunch: Sliced roast beef with one sliced avocado, handful of radishes and salad greens. Mayo for dipping of roast beef.

Dinner: Broiled salmon with broccoli in cheddar cheese.

Friday

Breakfast: 2 hard boiled eggs with slice of pan-fried ham, and ½ cup of raspberries and blackberries.

Lunch: Bacon wrapped mozzarella cheese sticks.

Dinner: Baked pork tenderloin with broccoli and asparagus.

Saturday

Breakfast: Bullet Coffee

Lunch: Can of sardines with an avocado.

Dinner: Spaghetti squash with meatballs in cheese sauce.

Week Three

Sunday

Breakfast: Guacamole and bacon.

Lunch: Smoked salmon, and cubed avocado with salad greens.

Dinner: Roast chicken with broccoli and cauliflower in cheddar cheese.

Monday

Breakfast: Chorizo sausage and 3 fried eggs.

Lunch: Smoked turkey wing with salad.

Dinner: NY Strip steak and salad.

Tuesday

Breakfast: Classic bacon and eggs with bullet coffee.

Lunch: Sliced deli turkey with full fat mayo, diced avocado, spinach in olive oil.

Dinner: Bell peppers stuffed with goat cheese and ground beef.

Wednesday

Breakfast: Scrambled eggs topped with guacamole with bullet coffee.

Lunch: Boiled shrimp, full fat mayo for dipping, three hard boiled eggs, on a bed of spinach drizzled in olive oil.

Dinner: Grilled Pork Sirloin Steaks with asparagus.

Thursday

Breakfast: Sausage and bacon 3-egg omelet.

Lunch: Shrimp and avocado spinach salad.

Dinner: Tilapia pan fried in butter with sautéed spinach.

Friday

Breakfast: Raspberries in heated coconut cream.

Lunch: Cauliflower pizza topped with pepperoni, mozzarella cheese, spinach, and white pizza sauce.

Dinner: Ribeye steak with salad.

Saturday

Breakfast: 2 breakfast sausages with 2 fried eggs.

Lunch: Bed of greens topped with avocados, tomatoes, onions, and canned sardines.

Dinner: Baked trout with sautéed spinach and broccoli.

Tuna with Spinach

Ingredients:

- ¼ cup olive oil
- 3 tuna steaks
- Salt and pepper to taste
- Red chile flakes to taste
- 2 teaspoons of lime juice
- Tablespoon lemon juice

Instructions:

Combine olive oil, seasonings, lime juice, and lemon juice in a bowl. Pour over tuna steaks and marinate for 30 minutes. Grill tuna steaks or broil, cooking to desired doneness. Prepare a bed of spinach on serving plates. Drizzle with lemon juice and olive oil. When tuna is done, place on top of spinach and serve.

Chicken Breasts with Mozzarella Cheese and Bacon

Ingredients:
4 slices thick-cut bacon
1 1/2 c. shredded mozzarella
4 boneless skinless chicken breasts Kosher salt
2 tsp. ranch seasoning
Ground black pepper
Chopped chives

Instructions:
Season chicken with ranch seasoning and black pepper. Preheat pan over medium heat. Cook strips of bacon, remove and set aside. Place chicken in bacon grease and cook until golden, about 5 minutes per side. Reduce heat to medium and add rest of ingredients, cover and cook for five minutes. While chicken is cooking, chop up bacon. Remove chicken from heat and allow to cool, then add to serving plates and top with

chopped bacon. Can be served with asparagus or sautéed spinach.

Keto meatloaf

Ingredients:

- 2 eggs
- ½ cup almond flour
- 2 pounds ground beef
- 1 chopped onion
- 1 chopped stalk of celery
- ¼ cup grated parmesan cheese
- 3 cloves minced garlic
- 1 cup shredded cheddar cheese
- 1 tablespoon soy sauce
- 1 teaspoon chili powder
- 1 teaspoon chopped oregano
- 8 strips of thick bacon
- Salt and pepper

Instructions:

Preheat over to 400. Heat skillet over medium, add 2 tablespoons olive oil. Add chopped onion and celery and cook until golden. Stir in garlic, chili powder and oregano. Cook for another minute. Remove from heat and add to a large bowl with ground beef, cheese, eggs, and remaining items. Mix together thoroughly, shape as desired, then place in a baking dish. Cover with strips of bacon. Cover baking dish with foil and bake for one hour.

Garlic Tilapia

Ingredients:

- 4 Tilapia filets
- 2 tablespoons extra virgin olive oil
- 3 cloves minced garlic
- 1 sliced lemon
- 1 tablespoon chopped or dried parsley
- Juice and zest of one lemon
- 1 pound of asparagus
- salt and pepper to taste
- 3 tablespoons of butter

Instructions:

Preheat skillet over medium heat. Add tablespoon of butter and olive oil. Season tilapia to taste, then cook in plan for 5 minutes per side. Remove from heat, and add more olive oil. Cook asparagus until done, seasoning as desired. Add 2 more tablespoons of butter with garlic, then return tilapia to pan and cook for a minute to allow garlic flavor to infuse the fish. Remove from heat and add to serving plates, drizzling with lemon as desired.

Conclusion

Thanks for reading Keto Diet 2020. I hope that this book has met the main goal we set out to achieve, in that it has given you a basic education about the keto diet. After finishing this book, you should understand what the keto diet is and why it works. You should know what the main benefits of the keto diet are. There should also be a basic understanding of the foods to eat and the foods to avoid, and also how to overcome problems on the keto diet.

The keto diet can help you overcome problems involving weight and health that you may have been dealing with for years. It can help you get more energy and feel better, while losing weight at the same time, all the while avoiding hunger.

The keto diet can also help you avoid problems like diabetes, cancer, and even heart disease.

Thank you again for reading this book, and if you have found the book to be useful, please leave a nice review for us!

Keto Diet Cookbook 2020

Ketogenic Diet Recipes Made Very Easy To Lose Weight + Special Menu Plan with Calorie Foods. Reduce Triglycerides & Burn Fat Forever

Elisa Baker

Introduction

Congratulations on purchasing *Keto Diet Cookbook 2020* and thank you for doing so.

The following chapters will discuss many ways to enjoy your day using delicious recipes to prepare your meals. Use your Air Fryer, slow cooker, crockpot, and ice cream maker to make the delicious treats. Your new cookbook will provide you with many new ways to change your lifestyle. You will never be hungry and will still remain within the constraints of the keto plan.

You must decide how you want to proceed with your diet plan. It is always best to discuss these essential steps with your physician. There are four methods, so you better understand the different levels of the keto diet plan. As a guideline, use these standards to stay within your chosen carbohydrate limits on the keto plan:

Method # 1: The standard ketogenic diet (SKD) elements are moderate protein, high-fat, and is low carbs. Generally, this diet is considered a low-carbohydrate (5% average), high-fat (75% average), and moderate protein (20% average) diet plan. (These counts and can vary.)

Method # 2: Workout times will call for the targeted keto diet or known by some as TKD. The process consists of adding additional carbohydrates to the diet plan during the times when you are more active. This is popular with sportsmen and women who are much more active.

Method # 3: The cyclical ketogenic diet (CKD) involves a restricted five-day keto diet plan followed by two high-carb days.

Method 4: The high-protein keto diet is comparable to the standard keto plan (SKD) in all aspects. However, you will consume more protein. Its ratio is repeatedly noted as maintaining 35% protein, 5%

carbs, and 60% fat. (Once again, these are average percentages.)

The Internet provides you with several ways to calculate your daily intake of carbs. Try an easy to follow <u>keto calculator</u> for assistance. Begin your weight loss process by making a habit of checking your levels when you want to know what essentials your body needs during the course of your dieting plan. You'll document your personal information such as height and weight. The Internet calculator will provide you with essential math.

The keto plan is used daily to provide you with many benefits. For example, you will achieve improved mental focus. Your brain is approximately <u>60% fat</u> by weight. By increasing your fatty food intake; you will have better focus. It can maintain itself and work at full capacity.

Let's Begin!

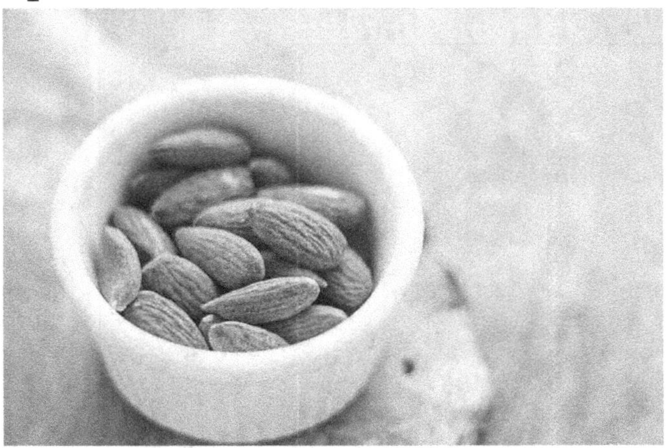

Almond - Coconut Egg Wraps

Yields Provided: 4 Servings
Nutritional Counts Per Serving:
- **Calories**: 111
- **Net Carbs**: 3 g
- **Total Fat Content**: 7.5 g
- **Protein**: 8 g

Ingredients Needed:
- Eggs (5)
- Coconut flour (1 tbsp.)
- Sea salt (.25 tsp.)
- Almond meal (2 tbsp.)

How to Prepare:
1. Measure and add the fixings into a blender and work until creamy.
2. Warm a skillet using the med-high temperature setting.
3. Pour 2 tbsp. of batter into the pan and cook for three minutes.
4. Flip it over and continue cooking for another three minutes.
5. Serve hot.

Avocado & Bacon Omelet

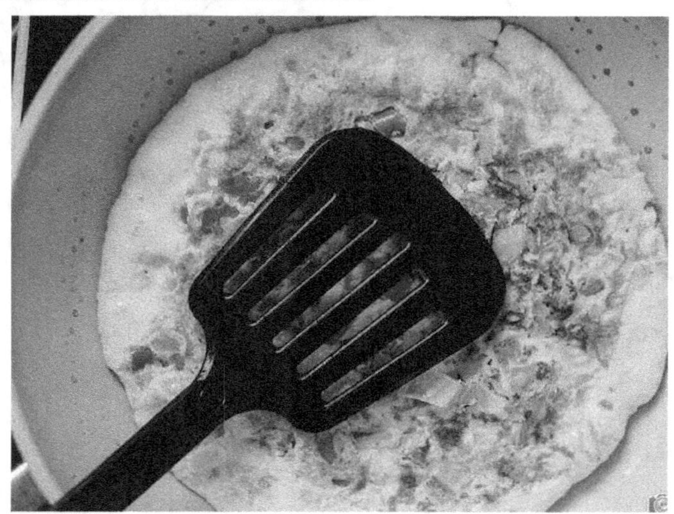

Yields Provided: 1 Serving
Nutritional Counts Per Serving:
- **Calories**: 719
- **Net Carbs**: 3.3 g
- **Total Fat Content**: 63 g
- **Protein**: 30 g

Ingredients Needed:
- Crispy bacon (1 slice)
- Large eggs (2)
- Freshly grated parmesan cheese (.5 cup)
- Ghee or coconut oil or butter (2 tbsp.)
- Salt (1 pinch)
- Avocado (.5 of 1 small)

How to Prepare:
1. Prepare the bacon to your liking, and set aside.
2. Combine the eggs, parmesan cheese and your choice of finely chopped herbs.
3. Heat a skillet and add the butter to melt using the med-high

heat setting.

4. When the pan is hot, whisk and add the eggs.

5. Prepare the omelet working it towards the middle of the pan for about 30 seconds. When firm, flip and cook for another 30 seconds.

6. Arrange on a plate and garnish with the crunched bacon bits. Serve with sliced avocado.

Bacon Hash

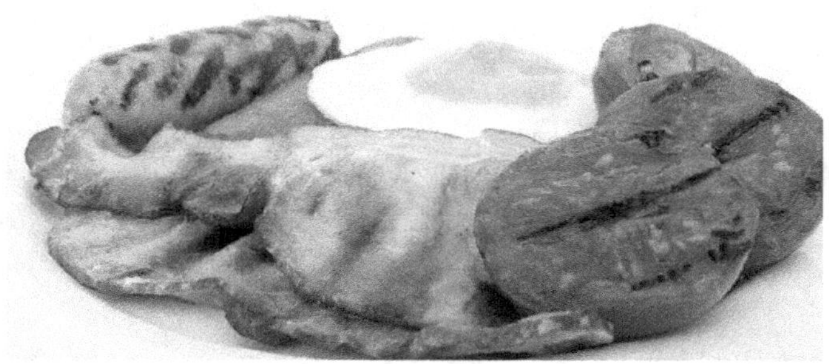

Yields Provided: 2 Servings
Nutritional Counts Per Serving:
- **Calories**: 366
- **Net Carbs**: 9 g
- **Total Fat Content**: 24 g
- **Protein**: 23 g

Ingredients Needed:
- Bacon slices (6)
- Small onion (1)
- Small green pepper (1)
- Jalapeños (2)
- Eggs (4)

How to Prepare:
1. Chop the bacon into chunks using a food processor. Set aside for now.
2. Thinly slice the onions and peppers into thin strips. Dice the jalapeños as small as possible.
3. Warm a skillet and fry the veggies.
4. Once browned, combine the fixings and cook until crispy.
5. Place on a serving dish with the eggs.

Bagels with Cheese

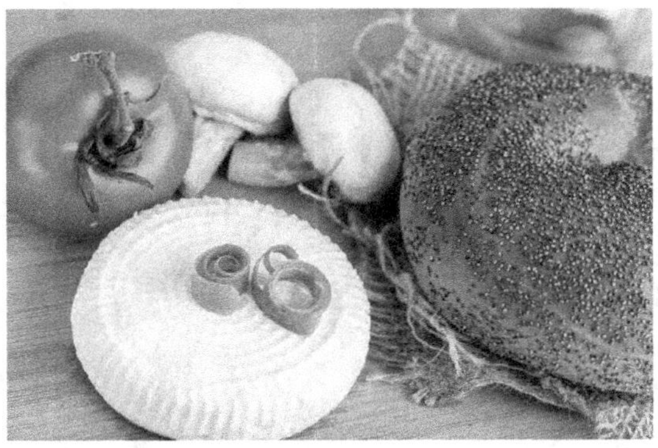

Yields Provided: 6 Servings
Nutritional Counts Per Serving:

- **Calories**: 374
- **Net Carbs**: 8 g
- **Total Fat Content**: 31 g
- **Protein**: 19 g

Ingredients Needed:

- Baking powder (1 tsp.)
- Cream cheese (3 oz.)
- Almond flour (1.5 cups)
- Shredded mozzarella cheese (2.5 cups)
- Eggs (2)

How to Prepare:

1. Combine the baking powder, mozzarella, flour, and cream cheese in a mixing container. Pop into the microwave for about one minute. Mix well.
2. Let the mixture cool and add the eggs. Break apart into six sections and shape into round bagels.
3. *Note*: You can also sprinkle with a seasoning of your choice or pinch of salt if desired.
4. Bake until the edges of the bagels are golden brown (12 - 15

min.).

5. Cool and store.

Belgian Style Waffles

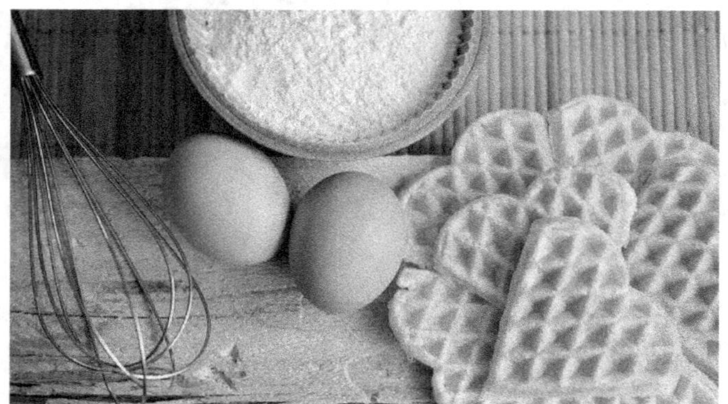

Yields Provided: 4 Servings
Nutritional Counts Per Serving:
- **Calories**: 247
- **Net Carbs**: 3 g
- **Total Fat Content**: 19 g
- **Protein**: 11 g

Ingredients Needed:
- Melted butter or ghee (4 tbsp.)
- Eggs (6)
- Salt (.5 tsp.)
- Bak. powder (.5 tsp.)
- Coconut flour (.33 cup)
- *Optional:* SweetLeaf stevia drops (.125 tsp.)

How to Prepare:
1. In a blender, mix the butter and eggs until incorporated.
2. Pour in the salt, stevia, and baking powder. Blend well to combine.
3. Fold in the flour and let it rest to thicken (5 min.)
4. If needed, pour in small amounts of water to thin the batter.
5. Prepare in the waffle maker and serve.

Blueberry Hemp Seed Breakfast Oatmeal

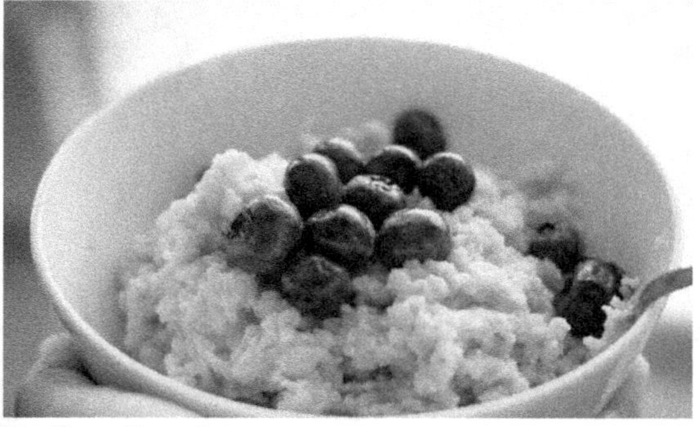

Yields Provided: 2 Servings
Nutritional Counts Per Serving:
- **Calories**: 436
- **Net Carbs**: 5 g
- **Protein**: 21 g
- **Total Fat Content**: 31 g

Ingredients Needed:
- Unsweetened almond milk/water (1 cup)
- Ground cinnamon (.5 tsp.)
- Hemp seed hearts (.5 cup)
- Flaxseed meal (.5 cup)
- Swerve (2 tbsp.)
- Unsweetened coconut flakes (1 tbsp.)
- Fresh blueberries (.25 cup)
- Vanilla extract (1 tsp.)
- Sliced almonds (1 tbsp.)

How to Prepare:
1. Place a saucepan over the med-high heat using the stovetop. Pour in the milk, vanilla extract, and cinnamon. Stir.
2. Toss in the hemp seed hearts and flaxseed meal. Change the temperature on the stove to medium heat.
3. Stir in the sweetener. Keep the mixture on the heat (uncovered) until the oatmeal thickens.

4. Serve in a bowl and top with almonds, blueberries, and other keto-friendly toppings.

Blueberry Ricotta Pancakes

Yields Provided: 5 Servings
Nutritional Counts Per Serving:
- **Calories**: 311
- **Net Carbs**: 6 g
- **Total Fat Content**: 23 g
- **Protein**: 15 g

Ingredients Needed:
- Large eggs (3)
- Vanilla extract (.5 tsp.)
- Unsweetened vanilla almond milk (.25 cup)
- Ricotta (.75 cup)
- Golden flaxseed meal (.5 cup)
- Salt (.25 tsp.)
- Baking powder (1 tsp.)
- Almond flour (1 cup)
- Stevia powder (.5 tsp.)
- Blueberries (.25 cup)
- *Optional:* Keto-friendly syrup of choice

How to Prepare:
1. Mix the eggs, milk, ricotta, and vanilla extract with an electric mixer.
2. Combine the baking powder, flaxseed meal, salt, flour, and stevia in another dish.
3. Slowly, combine the dry fixings into the blender to form the batter. Use two to three blueberries for each pancake.
4. Add the butter to a hot skillet using the medium heat setting. When it melts, add the batter using two tablespoons for each serving.
5. Serve or set aside to cool.

6. You can serve or freeze to use later if you have limited time. If you know your schedule will be rushed; you can pour the syrup in a cup with a top.

Brunch BLT Wrap

Yields Provided: 1 Serving
Nutritional Counts Per Serving:
- **Calories**: 256
- **Net Carbs**: 2 g
- **Total Fat Content**: 24 g
- **Protein**: 8 g

Ingredients Needed:
- Crispy fried bacon slices (4)
- Romaine or Iceberg lettuce leaves (2)
- Chopped tomatoes (.25 cup)
- Mayo (1 tbsp.)
- Pepper and salt (to your liking)

How to Prepare:
1. Spread the layer of mayonnaise on one side of the lettuce.
2. Add the bacon and tomato. Season to your liking. Roll it up and serve.

Brunch Tomato Pesto Mug Cake

Yields Provided: 1 Serving
Nutritional Counts Per Serving:
- **Calories**: 460
- **Net Carbs**: 4 g
- **Total Fat Content**: 45 g
- **Protein**: 13 g

Ingredients Needed:
- Large egg (1)
- Almond flour (2 tbsp.)
- Butter (2 tbsp.)
- Bak. powder (.5 tsp.)

Pesto Ingredients Needed:
- Almond flour (1 tbsp.)
- Sun-dried tomato pesto (5 tsp. or as desired)
- Salt (1 pinch)

How to Prepare:
1. Combine each of the fixings in a mug, but keep a little pesto for the garnish.
2. Microwave the cup for 70-80 seconds.
3. Lightly tap the mug on a serving dish. It will fall right out. Top the cake off with the pesto, and enjoy.

Cheesy Italian Omelet

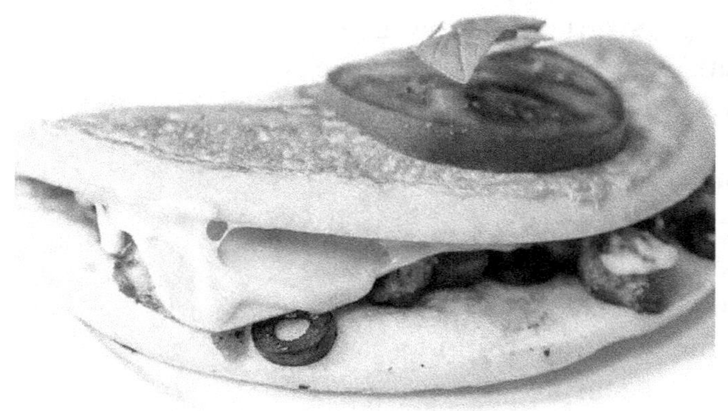

Yields Provided: 2 Servings
Nutritional Counts Per Serving:
- **Calories**: 451
- **Net Carbs**: 3 g
- **Total Fat Content**: 36 g
- **Protein**: 33 g

Ingredients Needed:
- Eggs (2)
- Water (1 tbsp.)
- Butter or ghee (1 tbsp.)
- Salami or prosciutto (3 thin slices)
- Basil (6 leaves)
- Mozzarella cheese slices (2 oz.)
- Tomato (5 thin slices)
- Pepper and salt (as desired)

How to Prepare:
1. Whisk the water and eggs together.
2. Toss the ghee/butter in a frying pan (med. setting) to melt. Whisk and pour in the eggs and cook for about 30 seconds.
3. Spread out the meat slices over top of the egg followed by the

cheese, tomatoes, and slices of basil. Give the mixture a shake of pepper and salt.

4. Cook approximately 2 minutes until firm. Flip, and continue cooking for another minute before folding in half. Cover the pan and simmer over low heat.

5. When the center is done, just add the omelet to a plate and serve.

Cocoa Waffles

Yields Provided: 5 Servings

Nutritional Counts Per Serving:

- **Calories**: 289
- **Net Carbs**: 3.4 g
- **Total Fat Content**: 27 g
- **Protein**: 7 g

Ingredients Needed:

- Separated eggs (5)
- Unsweetened cocoa (.25 cup)
- Granular sweetener (3 tbsp.)
- Coconut flour (4 tbsp.)
- Baking powder (1 tsp.)
- Melted butter (4.5 oz.)
- Milk of choice (3 tbsp.)
- Vanilla (1 tsp.)

How to Prepare:

1. Use a whisk to prepare the egg whites. Briskly mix to form stiff peaks.
2. In another container, whisk the sweetener, baking powder, and cocoa with the egg yolks.
3. Add the butter to the dry mixture. Stir in vanilla and milk.
4. Fold in the prepared egg whites a little at a time.
5. Transfer the mixture in the waffle maker.
6. Cook until they are golden brown.
7. Serve.

Cream Cheese Eggs

Yields Provided: 1 Serving
Nutritional Counts Per Serving:
- **Calories**: 341
- **Net Carbs**: 3 g
- **Total Fat Content**: 31 g
- **Protein**: 15 g

Ingredients Needed:
- Butter (1 tbsp.)
- Eggs (2)
- Soft cream cheese with chives (2 tbsp.)

How to Prepare:
1. Heat a skillet and melt the butter. Whisk the eggs with the cream cheese.
2. Add to the pan and stir until they're like you like them.

Creamy Basil Baked Sausage

Yields Provided: 12 Servings
Nutritional Counts Per Serving:
- **Calories:** 316
- **Net Carbs:** 4 g
- **Total Fat Content:** 23 g
- **Protein:** 23 g

Ingredients Needed:
- Italian sausage - pork/turkey or chicken (3 lb.)
- Cream cheese (8 oz.)
- Heavy cream (.25 cup)
- Basil pesto (.25 cup)
- Mozzarella (8 oz.)

How to Prepare:
1. Warm up the oven to reach 400° Fahrenheit.
2. Lightly spritz a casserole dish with cooking oil spray. Add the sausage to the dish and bake for 30 minutes.
3. Mix the heavy cream, pesto, and cream cheese.
4. Once the sauce is done, pour it over the casserole and top it off with a portion of cheese.
5. Bake for another 10 minutes. The sausage should reach 160° Fahrenheit in the center when checked with a meat thermometer.
6. *Option 2:* You can also broil for three minutes to brown the cheesy layer.

Eggs & Mackerel Brunch Plate

Yields Provided: 2 Servings
Nutritional Counts Per Serving:
- **Calories**: 689
- **Net Carbs**: 4 g
- **Total Fat Content**: 59 g
- **Protein**: 35 g

Ingredients Needed:
- Eggs (4)
- Butter for frying (2 tbsp.)
- Canned mackerel in tomato sauce (8 oz.)
- Lettuce (2 oz.)
- Red onion (.5 of 1)
- Olive oil (.25 cup)
- Black pepper & salt (to your liking)

How to Prepare:
1. Warm the frying pan and prepare your eggs in the butter.
2. Add lettuce to a platter and layer with the onion and mackerel.
3. Arrange the eggs to the side, adding a dusting of pepper and salt as desired.
4. Spritz the oil over the salad and serve.

Green Buttered Eggs

Yields Provided: 2 Servings
Nutritional Counts Per Serving:
- **Calories**: 311
- **Net Carbs**: 2.5 g
- **Total Fat Content**: 27.5 g
- **Protein**: 13 g

Ingredients Needed:
- Coconut oil (1 tbsp.)
- Organic butter (2 tbsp.)
- Cloves of garlic (2)
- Fresh cilantro (.5 cup)
- Fresh parsley (.5 cup)
- Fresh thyme leaves (1 tsp.)
- Organic eggs (4)
- Ground cayenne (.25 tsp.)
- Sea salt (.25 tsp.)
- Ground cumin (.25 tsp.)

How to Prepare:
1. Mince the garlic and finely chop the parsley and cilantro.
2. Heat a skillet and melt the oil and butter. Toss in the garlic. Sauté for three minutes (low setting). Sprinkle using the thyme. Sauté another 30 seconds.
3. Toss in the cilantro and parsley using the medium heat setting for about three more minutes.
4. Break in the eggs (don't break the yolk).
5. Cover and cook about four to six minutes until the yolks are set (runny yolk is three to four minutes).
6. Serve immediately.

Ham Cheese Soufflé

Yields Provided: 4 Servings
Nutritional Counts Per Serving:
- **Total Fat Content**: 38 g
- **Calories**: 460
- **Net Carbs**: 5 g
- **Protein**: 24 g

Ingredients Needed:
- Diced yellow onion (1 small)
- Minced garlic (2 cloves)
- Fresh chopped chives (2 tbsp.)
- Shredded cheddar cheese (1 cup)
- Heavy cream (.5 cup)
- Eggs (6 large)
- Diced ham (6 oz.)
- Salt and pepper (as desired)
- Olive oil (2 tbsp.)
- _Also Needed_: 6 oz. ramekins (4)

How to Prepare:
1. Program the oven setting to reach 400° Fahrenheit. Lightly grease the ramekins.
2. Use the medium heat temperature setting in a skillet on the stovetop to warm the oil.
3. Toss in the onions to sauté for five minutes. Next, toss in the garlic and sauté for one more minute.
4. Whisk together the rest of the fixings in a mixing bowl.
5. Add the cooked onions and garlic. Stir well, then divide among the ramekins.
6. Bake until the egg is cooked through (18 to 22 minutes).
7. Cool slightly before serving.

Lemon Waffles

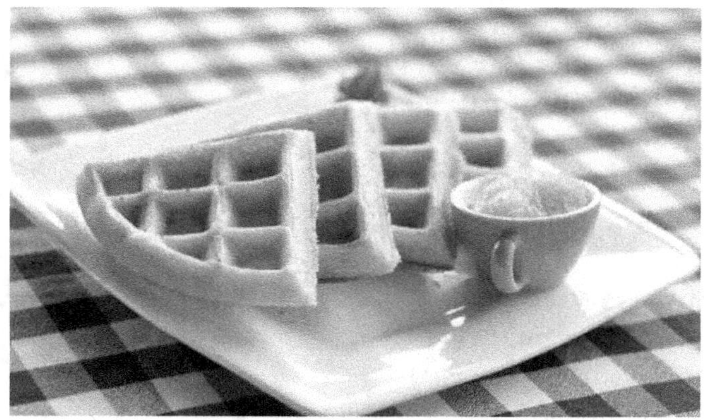

Yields Provided: 4 Servings

Nutritional Counts Per Serving:

- **Calories**: 99
- **Net Carbs**: 1.8 g
- **Total Fat Content**: 8.2 g
- **Protein**: 1.1 g

Ingredients Needed:

- Coconut flour (.25 cup)
- Whole psyllium husks (1 tbsp.)
- Salt (1 pinch)
- Baking powder (.5 tsp.)
- Melted coconut oil (1.5 tbsp.) or Melted coconut butter (2 tbsp.)
- Granulated sweetener (1 tbsp.)
- Lemon juice (1 tbsp.)
- Nondairy milk of choice (5 tbsp.)
- Vanilla extract (.5 tsp.)

How to Prepare:

1. Warm a cast-iron pan or ceramic non-stick pan using the med-low heat setting. Grease the pan with additional coconut oil as needed.

2. Whisk the coconut flour, psyllium, baking powder, and salt.

3. Combine with the rest of the fixings in another container.

4. Stir the dry fixings into the wet ones until thoroughly mixed. Let it rest until a stiff dough forms, about 3 to 5 minutes, molding with your hands.

5. Tip: If the coconut oil and psyllium do not absorb enough liquid to form the dough, stir in an additional tablespoon of coconut flour.

6. Divide and shape into four dough balls.

7. Flatten the balls and cook for approximately five minutes per side, until golden.

8. Let cool for a minute or so before topping.

Pumpkin Spice Waffles

Yields Provided: 2 Servings
Nutritional Counts Per Serving:
- **Total Fat Content**: 25 g
- **Calories**: 290
- **Net Carbs**: 5 g
- **Protein**: 14 g

Ingredients Needed:
- Coconut milk (.33 cup)
- Vanilla extract (1 tsp.)
- Liquid stevia (7 drops)
- Canned pumpkin (.25 cup)
- Large eggs (2)
- Swerve sweetener (3 tbsp.)
- Baking powder (1 tsp.)
- Flaxseed meal (2 tbsp.
- Almond flour (.5 cup)
- Pumpkin pie spice (1.5 tsp.)
- Coconut spray (spritz as needed)

How to Prepare:
1. Grease and warm the waffle iron. Whip each of the wet fixings in a mixing container.
2. Combine the dry components using a sifter or whisk. Sift them into the wet ones as you go. Mix well.
3. Pour in the batter. Serve while they're hot with a favorite fruit or syrup (add the carbs).

Sausage Hot Pockets

Yields Provided: 2 Servings
Nutritional Counts Per Serving:
- **Calories**: 510
- **Net Carbs**: 6.6 g
- **Total Fat Content**: 41.4 g
- **Protein**: 26.3 g

Ingredients Needed:
- Low-moisture shredded mozzarella cheese (.75 cup)
- Almond flour (.33 cup)
- Egg white (1)
- _Optional:_ Xanthan gum (.5 tsp.)

Ingredients Needed - The Filling:
- Shredded Mexican blend cheese
- Avocado oil (1 tbsp.)
- Large eggs (2)
- Kiolbassa Jalapeño Smoked Sausage (1)
- Bell pepper (2 tbsp.)
- Jalapeño pepper (1 tbsp.)
- Onion (2 tbsp.)

How to Prepare:
1. Heat the oven to reach 400° Fahrenheit.
2. Melt the cheese in the microwave for about 30 seconds.
3. Stir in the rest of the fixings. Roll into a ball, kneading one or two times.
4. Place between two sheets of parchment baking paper. With a rolling pin, prepare the dough to a .25-inch thickness.
5. Warm oil in a cast-iron skillet using the med-high heat setting.
6. Once it is hot; add in onions and peppers to simmer for two or three minutes until softened.
7. Stir in the sausage, cooking for another 2 to 3 minutes. Push

aside, and add the eggs. Scramble until done.

8. Place the mixture into the center of the dough. Tuck in each of the sides until fully enclosed. Poke with a fork for the steam to escape.

9. Bake for 20 minutes. Remove and slice in half to serve.

Delicious Coffee & Other Breakfast Beverages

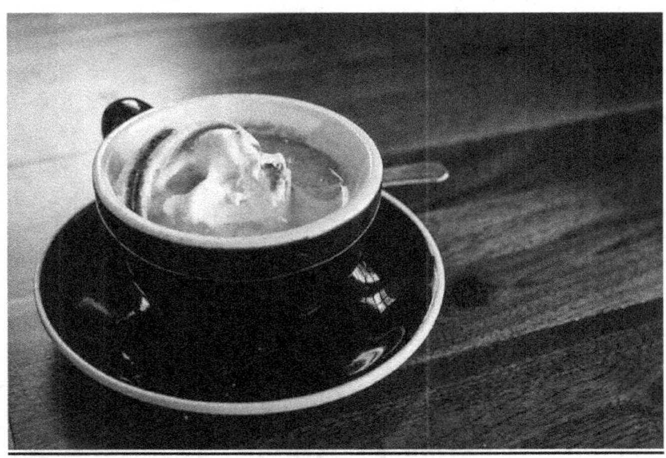

Yields Provided: 1 Serving
Nutritional Counts Per Serving:
- **Calories**: 320
- **Net Carbs**: 0 g
- **Total Fat Content**: 51 g
- **Protein**: 1 g

Ingredients Needed:
- MCT oil powder (2 tbsp.)
- Ghee or butter (2 tbsp.)
- Hot coffee (1.5 cups)

How to Prepare:
1. Pour the hot coffee into your blender.
2. Measure and add the powder and butter. Blend until frothy.
3. Serve using a large mug.

Coffee & Cream

Yields Provided: 1 Serving
Nutritional Counts Per Serving:
- **Calories**: 206
- **Net Carbs**: 2 g
- **Total Fat Content**: 22 g
- **Protein**: 2 g

Ingredients Needed:
- Brewed coffee (.75 cup)
- Heavy whipping cream (4 tbsp.)

How to Prepare:
1. Make your coffee as desired.
2. Add the cream in a saucepan and simmer until it's frothy.
3. Pour the cream into the cup and gently stir.
4. Serve with a slice of cheese or a portion of nuts at any time.

Dairy-Free Keto Latte

Yields Provided: 2 Servings
Nutritional Counts Per Serving:
- **Calories**: 191
- **Net Carbs**: 1 g
- **Total Fat Content**: 18 g
- **Protein**: 6 g

Ingredients Needed:
- Eggs (2)
- Boiling water (1.5 cups)
- Coconut oil (2 tbsp.)
- Vanilla extract (1 pinch)
- Ground ginger or pumpkin pie spice (1 tsp.)

How to Prepare:
1. Combine all of the fixings in the blender.
2. Serve right away.

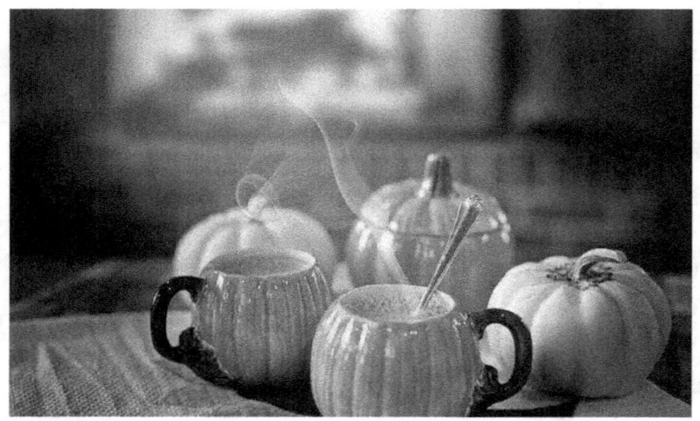

Yields Provided: 1 Serving
Nutritional Counts Per Serving:
- **Calories**: 216
- **Net Carbs**: 1 g
- **Total Fat Content**: 23 g
- **Protein**: 0.5 g

Ingredients Needed:
- Instant coffee powder (1.5 - 2 tsp.)
- Boiling water (1 cup)
- Pumpkin pie spice or cinnamon (1 tsp.)
- Unsalted butter (1 oz.)
- *Also Needed*: Immersion Blender

How to Prepare:
1. Combine the instant coffee, spices, and butter in a mixing dish.
2. Pour in the water and blend for 20 to 30 seconds until foamy.
3. Pour into the cup and sprinkle with the spice.
4. Serve with a dollop of whipped cream if desired.

Vanilla Coffee with Whipped Cream

Yields Provided: 1 Serving
Nutritional Counts Per Serving:
- **Calories**: 206
- **Net Carbs**: 2 g
- **Total Fat Content**: 21 g
- **Protein**: 2 g

Ingredients Needed:
- Coffee (1 cup prepared)
- Heavy whipping cream (.25 cup)
- Vanilla extract (.25 tsp.)
- _Optional Garnishes:_ Ground cinnamon & Cocoa powder

How to Prepare:
1. Prepare your coffee as you normally do without the extras.
2. Whip the cream with the vanilla to form soft peaks.
3. Pour the coffee into a large mug with a dollop of cream.
4. Sprinkle with a dusting of cinnamon or cocoa powder to your liking.
5. Serve.

Wintery Hot Chocolate

Yields Provided: 1 Serving

Nutritional Counts Per Serving:
- **Calories**: 216
- **Net Carbs**: 1 g
- **Total Fat Content**: 23 g
- **Protein**: 1 g

Ingredients Needed:
- Cocoa powder (1 tbsp.)
- Unsalted butter (1 oz.)
- Vanilla extract (.25 tsp.)
- Boiling water (1 cup)
- *Optional:* Powdered erythritol (1 tsp.)
- *Also Needed:* Immersion blender

How to Prepare:
1. Add each of the fixings into a tall container to prepare using the blender.
2. Blend for 15 to 20 seconds until the foam is no longer on the top.
3. Pour the cocoa and serve.

Avocado - Corn Salad

Yields Provided: 4 Servings
Nutritional Counts Per Serving:
- **Calories**: 147
- **Net Carbs**: 4.5 g
- **Total Fat Content**: 11 g
- **Protein**: 3.5 g

Ingredients Needed - The Salad:
- Cooked - corn on the cob - husk removed (1)
- Romaine head (1 chopped)
- Quartered grape tomatoes (4)
- Sliced red onion (.25 cup)
- Sliced avocado (.5 of 1)

Ingredients Needed - The Dressing:
- Minced shallots (1 tbsp.)
- White wine vinegar (2 tbsp.)
- Dijon mustard (2 tsp.)
- 1% Vegan buttermilk (6 tbsp.)
- Garlic powder (.25 tsp.)
- Black pepper (1 pinch)
- Kosher salt (.5 tsp.)
- Extra-virgin olive oil (2 tbsp.)

How to Prepare:
1. Whisk each of the dressing components and pour them into a serving jar.
2. Combine the salad fixings in a large salad bowl and toss using the dressing.

Caprese Salad

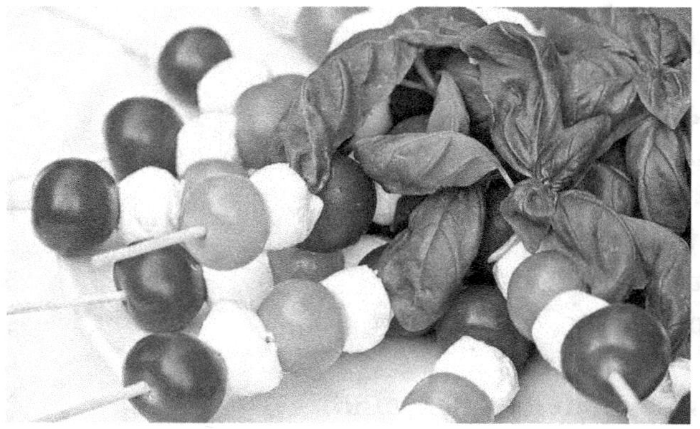

Yields Provided: 4 Servings
Nutritional Counts Per Serving:
- **Calories**: 191
- **Total Fat Content**: 64 g
- **Net Carbs**: 5 g
- **Protein**: 8 g

Ingredients Needed:
- Grape tomatoes (3 cups)
- Peeled garlic cloves (4)
- Avocado oil (2 tbsp.)
- Mozzarella balls (19 pearl-sized)
- Baby spinach leaves (4 cups)
- Brine reserved from the cheese (1 tbsp.)
- Pesto (1 tbsp.)
- Fresh basil leaves (.25 cup)

How to Prepare:
1. Use a layer of foil to line a baking tray.
2. Set the oven temperature setting to 400° Fahrenheit.
3. Arrange the cloves and tomatoes on the baking pan and drizzle using the oil. Bake until the tops are lightly browned (20-30 min.).

4. Drain the liquid from the mozzarella (saving one tablespoon). Mix the pesto with the brine.
5. Rinse and drain the spinach before adding to a large salad bowl. Transfer the tomatoes to the dish along with the roasted garlic. Drizzle with the pesto sauce.
6. Garnish with the mozzarella balls and freshly torn basil leaves.

Chicken-Pecan Salad & Cucumber Bites

Yields Provided: 2 Servings
Nutritional Counts Per Serving:
- **Calories**: 323
- **Net Carbs**: 3 g
- **Total Fat Content**: 24 g
- **Protein**: 23 g

Ingredients Needed:
- Cucumber (1)
- Precooked chicken breast (1 cup)
- Celery (.25 cup)
- Mayonnaise (2 tbsp.)
- Pecans (.25 cup)
- Himalayan Pink salt & Black pepper (1 pinch of ea.)

How to Prepare:
1. Peel and slice the cucumber into .25-inch slices. Dice the chicken and celery. Chop the pecans. Combine the pecans, chicken, mayonnaise, and celery in a salad bowl. Sprinkle with pepper and salt.
2. Layout the cucumber slices and add a pinch of salt. Layer each one with a spoonful of the chicken salad. Serve.

Cobb Salad

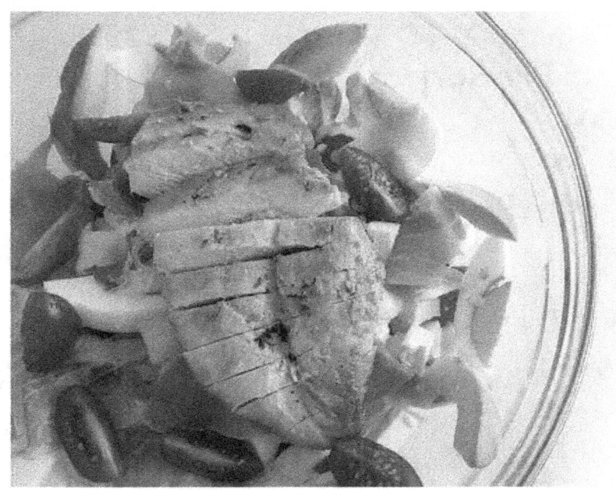

Yields Provided: 2 Servings
Nutritional Counts Per Serving:
- **Calories**: 600
- **Net Carbs**: 3 g
- **Total Fat Content**: 48 g
- **Protein**: 43 g

Ingredients Needed:
- Bacon strips (2)
- Hard-boiled egg (1)
- Spinach (1 cup)
- Campari tomato (.5 of 1)
- Chicken breast (2 oz.)
- Avocado (.25 of 1)
- Olive oil (1 tbsp.)
- White vinegar (.5 tsp.)

How to Prepare:
1. Cook the bacon and chicken. Shred or slice the chicken.
2. Cut all of the fixings into small pieces. Toss them to a bowl with the vinegar and oil. Toss gently and serve.

Greek Salad

Yields Provided: 1 Serving
Nutritional Counts Per Serving:
- **Calories**: 594
- **Net Carbs**: 8 g
- **Total Fat Content**: 58 g
- **Protein**: 12 g

Ingredients Needed:
- Tomato (.25 cup)
- Bell pepper (.25 cup)
- Olives (1 tbsp.)
- Red onion (.25 cup)
- Cucumber (.25 cup)
- Olive oil (3 tbsp.)
- Feta cheese (.5 cup)
- Red wine vinegar (.5 tbsp.)
- Black pepper and salt (as desired)

How to Prepare:
1. Dice the tomato, chop the olives, and slice the onion, cucumber, and pepper. Combine the bell pepper, tomato, cucumber, crumbled feta cheese, and onion.
2. Spritz using the oil and vinegar with a shake of pepper and salt to your liking.
3. Toss until all of the fixings are well mixed before serving.

Grilled Chicken Salad

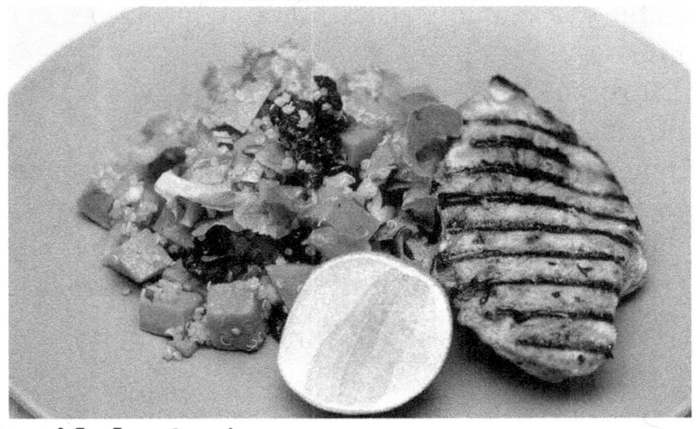

Yields Provided: 2 Servings
Nutritional Counts Per Serving:
- **Calories**: 187
- **Net Carbs**: 0.8 g
- **Total Fat Content**: 14 g
- **Protein**: 12 g

Ingredients Needed:
- Olive oil (1 tbsp.)
- Chicken thighs (2)
- Romaine lettuce (1 cup)
- Bacon (1 slice)
- Oregano (.5 tsp.)
- Pepper & Salt (.5 tsp. each)
- Parmesan cheese (2 tbsp.)

Ingredients Needed - For the Dressing:
- Lemon juice (1 tsp.)
- Mayonnaise (2 tbsp.)
- Dijon mustard (1 tbsp.)

How to Prepare:
1. Set the oven temperature at 355° Fahrenheit.

2. Arrange the chicken thighs on a baking tin. Sprinkle with oregano, olive oil, salt, and pepper.
3. Bake the chicken until cooked thoroughly or for approximately 15 minutes.
4. Either fry the bacon in a skillet or in the oven with the chicken until crispy or five to ten minutes.
5. Combine the mayonnaise, lemon juice, and mustard.
6. Transfer the cooked chicken to a cutting surface when cooled slightly. Slice into strips. Crunch the bacon to bits.
7. Prepare the salad and add the dressing. Add the sliced chicken and bacon, seasoning with parmesan cheese.

Jar Salad with Tempeh - Vegan

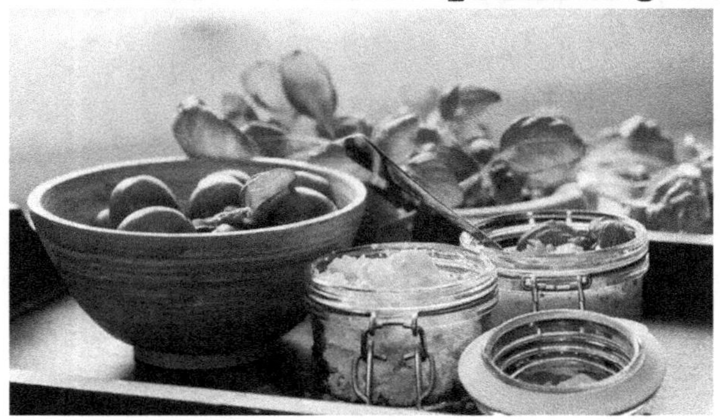

Yields Provided: 1 Serving
Nutritional Counts Per Serving:
- **Calories**: 215
- **Net Carbs**: 4 g
- **Total Fat Content**: 19 g
- **Protein**: 8 g

Ingredients Needed:
- Black pepper & salt (as desired)
- Keto-friendly mayonnaise (4 tbsp.)
- Scallion (.5)
- Cucumber (.25 oz.)
- Red bell pepper (.25 oz.)
- Cherry tomatoes (.25 oz.)
- Leafy greens (.25 oz.)
- Seasoned tempeh (4 oz.)

How to Prepare:
1. Chop or shred the vegetables as desired. Layer in the dark leafy greens first, followed by the onions, tomatoes, bell peppers, avocado, and shredded carrot.
2. Top the veggies off with the tempeh or use the same amount of another high-protein option to mix things up in later weeks.
3. Top with keto-vegan mayonnaise prior to serving.

Keto Salad Niçoise

Yields Provided: 1 Serving
Nutritional Counts Per Serving:
- **Calories**: 544
- **Net Carbs**: 8 g
- **Total Fat Content**: 48 g
- **Protein**: 18 g

Ingredients Needed:
- Large egg (1)
- Green onion (.5 tbsp.)
- Olives (.5 tbsp.)
- Celery (.5 cup)
- Snow peas (.5 cup)
- Olive oil (2 tbsp.)
- Garlic (.25 tbsp.)
- Romaine lettuce (1 cup)
- Crumbled feta cheese (.5 cup)
- Balsamic vinegar (1 tbsp.)

How to Prepare:
1. Hard boil the egg and remove the peel when cooled.
2. Chop the garlic, onion, celery, and olives.
3. Pour the olive oil into a small pan. Sauté the garlic, olives, and snow peas until the peas are bright green.
4. Prepare a large salad bowl and add the cooked veggies, shredded lettuce, celery, and green onion.
5. Make the dressing by whisking the vinegar, oil, salt, and pepper.
6. Combine the fixings and toss well before serving.

King-Sized Keto Salad

Yields Provided: 2 Servings
Nutritional Counts Per Serving:
- **Calories**: 581
- **Net Carbs**: 9 g
- **Total Fat Content**: 43 g
- **Protein**: 38 g

Ingredients Needed:
- Boneless breasts of chicken (2)
- Sliced avocado (1)
- Thinly cut bacon slices (6)
- Mixed leafy greens – your favorites (4 cups)
- Keto ranch dressing (4 tbsp.)

How to Prepare:
1. Heat the oven at 400° Fahrenheit.
2. Melt the ghee in a frying pan. Arrange the chicken in the pan – skin-side down. Prepare 5-6 minutes. Flip and cook about 30 more seconds.
3. Put the skillet in the oven. Roast for 10 to15 minutes. The internal temperature should reach 165° Fahrenheit.
4. Prepare a baking tin with a layer of parchment baking paper. Arrange the bacon slices on the tin and bake until crispy (10 min.).
5. Slice the chicken and avocado. Assemble the salad, beginning with the greens, avocado, chicken, and bacon.
6. Serve with a couple of tablespoons of dressing.

Pan-Fried Peach Scallops Salad

Yields Provided: 2 Servings
Nutritional Counts Per Serving:
- **Calories:** 130
- **Net Carbs:** 7 g
- **Total Fat Content:** 8 g
- **Protein:** 48 g

Ingredients Needed:
- Coconut oil for the pan
- Small scallops (1 dozen)
- Sliced peach (1)
- Sliced onion (.5 of 1)
- Oil (1 tsp.)
- Lemon juice (1 tsp.)
- Arugula leaves (5 oz.)

How to Prepare:
1. Warm the oil in a pan. Toss in the scallops. Sauté for about 5 minutes per side.
2. Fold in the arugula, onion slices, peaches, juice, and oil together well.
3. When ready to serve, add the scallops on top of the mixture.

Salad Sandwiches

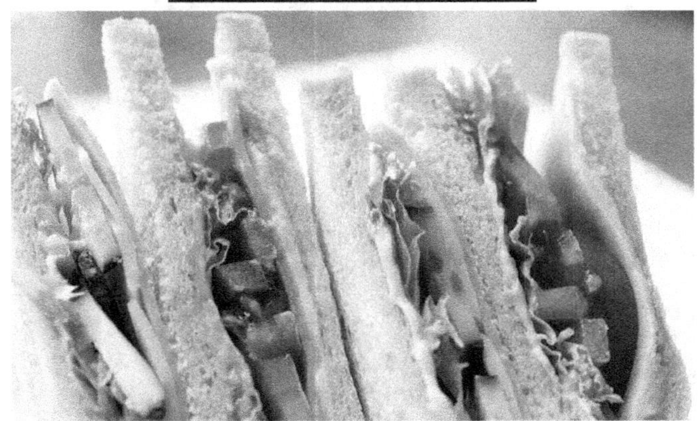

Yields Provided: 1 Serving

Nutritional Counts Per Serving:
- **Calories**: 374
- **Net Carbs**: 3 g
- **Total Fat Content**: 34 g
- **Protein**: 10 g

Ingredients Needed:
- Romaine lettuce (2 oz.)
- Butter (.5 oz.)
- Edam or your favorite cheese (1 oz.)
- Cherry tomato (1)
- Avocado (.5 of 1)

How to Prepare:
1. Rinse the lettuce. Drain in a colander.
2. Toss the lettuce to a salad dish and smear with the butter, cheese, avocado slices, and tomato on top.
3. Serve any time for a delicious meal or snack.

Shrimp Avocado Salad with Tomatoes & Feta

Yields Provided: 2 Servings
Nutritional Counts Per Serving:
- **Calories**: 430
- **Net Carbs**: 6.5 g
- **Total Fat Content**: 33 g
- **Protein**: 24 g

Ingredients Needed:
- Shrimp (8 oz.)
- Large avocado (1 diced)
- Beefsteak tomato (1 small)
- Feta cheese (.33 cup)
- Lemon juice (1 tbsp.)
- Cilantro/parsley (.33 cup)
- Olive oil (1 tbsp.)
- Melted salted butter (2 tbsp.)
- Freshly cracked black pepper & salt (.25 tsp. each)

How to Prepare:
1. Devein the shrimp, peel, and pat dry. Dice and drain the tomato, chop the parsley, and crumble the feta.
2. Melt the butter and toss the shrimp in a bowl until well-coated.
3. Warm a pan using the med-high heat setting until hot.
4. Toss the shrimp into the pan in a single layer, searing until it starts to become pink around the edges (1 min.). Flip and cook until the shrimp are cooked through (30 sec. approx.).
5. Transfer the shrimp to a plate to cool.
6. Add all other fixings into a large mixing bowl (diced tomato, diced avocado, lemon juice, olive oil, feta cheese, cilantro, pepper, and salt). Toss to mix.
7. Toss it together to serve.

Tuna Salad & Chives

Yields Provided: 4 Servings
Nutritional Counts Per Serving:
- **Calories**: 235
- **Net Carbs**: 1 g
- **Total Fat Content**: 18 g
- **Protein**: 20 g

Ingredients Needed:
- Tuna in olive oil (15 oz.)
- Chives (2 tbsp.)
- Mayonnaise (6 tbsp.)
- Pepper (.25 tsp.)
- Salt (to your liking)

How to Prepare:
1. Drain the tuna and finely chop the chives.
2. Add all of the fixings except the lettuce into a mixing bowl.
3. Toss well. Enjoy as-is or spoon into romaine lettuce leaves.

Vegetarian Club Salad

Yields Provided: 3 Servings
Nutritional Counts Per Serving:
- **Calories:** 330
- **Protein:** 17 g
- **Net Carbs:** 5 g
- **Total Fat Content:** 26 g

Ingredients Needed:
- Mayonnaise (2 tbsp.)
- Sour cream (2 tbsp.)
- Garlic powder (.5 tsp.)
- Dried parsley (1 tsp.)
- Onion powder (.5 tsp.)
- Milk (1 tbsp.)
- Dijon mustard (1 tbsp.)
- Large hard-boiled eggs (3)
- Cheddar cheese (4 oz.)
- Cherry tomatoes (.5 cup)
- Diced cucumber (1 cup)
- Torn romaine lettuce (3 cups)

How to Prepare:
1. Slice the hard-boiled eggs and cube the cheese. Cut the tomatoes into halves and dice the cucumber. Place the containers to the side for now.
2. Prepare the dressing (dried herbs, mayo, and sour cream) mixing well.
3. Add one tablespoon of milk to the mixture - and another if it's too thick.
4. Layer the salad - starting with the veggies, adding the cheese, and egg slices. Scoop a spoonful of mustard in the center along with a drizzle of dressing.
5. Toss and serve.

6. *Notes:* The nutritional counts are based on 2 tbsp. dressing.

Chapter 3: Lunch: Favorite Soups

Beef Cabbage Soup

Yields Provided: 8 Servings
Nutritional Counts Per Serving:
- **Calories**: 177
- **Net Carbs**: 4 g
- **Total Fat Content**: 11 g
- **Protein**: 12 g

Ingredients Needed:
- Olive oil (2 tbsp.)
- Onion (1 large)
- Ribeye fillet steak (1 lb.)
- Celery (1 stalk)
- Carrots (2 large)
- Green cabbage (1 small)
- Garlic (4 cloves)
- Beef stock/broth (6 cups)
- Fresh chopped parsley (3 tbsp. + more for serving)
- Dried thyme /rosemary/ basil & oregano (2 tsp. each or to your liking)
- Onion/garlic powder (2 tsp.)
- Freshly-cracked black pepper & salt (as desired)

How to Prepare:
1. Mince the garlic and chop the onion, celery, and carrots. Chop the cabbage into bite-sized chunks. Trim the steak of all visible fat. Chop into one-inch chunks.
2. Warm oil in a large pot using the medium heat temperature setting.
3. Toss in the cut meat. Sear until browned. Toss in the onions

and sauté until transparent (3-4 min.).

4. Toss in the celery and carrots, mixing well for about 3-4 minutes.

5. Fold in the cabbage and sauté an additional five minutes. Toss in the garlic, and sauté for another minute, mixing all fixings through.

6. Pour in the stock/broth, dried herbs, parsley, and onion or garlic powder, mixing well. Simmer and reduce the heat to med-low. Cover with a top.

7. Simmer until the cabbage and carrots are softened (10 to 15 min.). Toss the salt, pepper, and extra dried herbs, as desired. Serve warm.

Broccoli Curry Soup

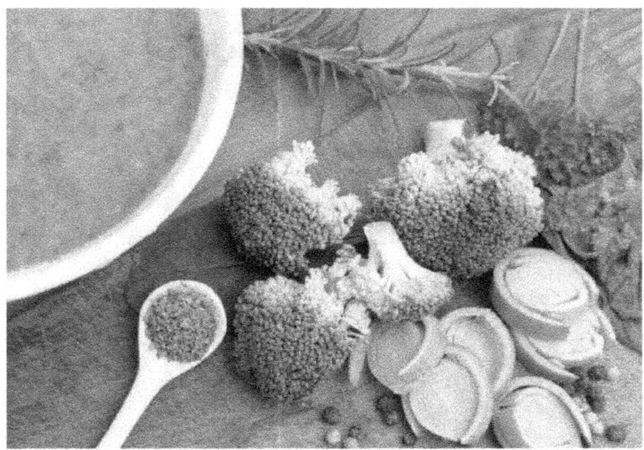

Yields Provided: 4 Servings

Nutritional Counts Per Serving:
- **Calories**: 375
- **Total Fat Content**: 20 g
- **Net Carbs**: 5 g
- **Protein**: 17 g

Ingredients Needed:
- Salt & Black pepper (as needed)
- Onion (1 chopped)
- Curry (1 tbsp.)
- Coconut oil (2 tbsp.)
- Vegetable stock (1 liter)
- Coconut cream (1 cup)
- Cheese substitute - your choice (75 g grated)
- Broccoli (1 lb.)

How to Prepare:
1. Pour coconut oil into a frying pan on the stovetop using the med-high heat setting.
2. Mix in the onion. Simmer for approximately six minutes.
3. Lower the temperature to medium. Then, add in the broth until it begins to simmer. Mix in the broccoli as well as any

seasonings before adding curry. Simmer for 20 minutes.
4.   Pour into a blender before mixing in the cheese substitute.
5.   Blend well.

Chicken Cauliflower Rice Soup

Yields Provided: 6 Servings
Nutritional Counts Per Serving:
- **Calories**: 286
- **Net Carbs**: 7 g
- **Total Fat Content**: 25 g
- **Protein**: 7 g

Ingredients Needed:
- Ghee or olive oil (2 tbsp.)
- Onion (1 small)
- Carrots (2 peeled)
- Celery (2 stalks)
- Bay leaf (1)
- Pepper & salt (as desired)
- Fresh thyme (1 tsp.)
- Chicken stock/broth (4 cups)
- Canned coconut milk - full fat (2 cups)
- Chicken breast (1)
- Cauliflower rice (2 cups)
- Fresh flat-leaf parsley (.25 cup)

How to Prepare:
1.   Chop or dice the carrots, celery, and onions. Discard the skin and bones from the chicken.
2.   Melt the ghee or pour the oil into a large soup pot. Toss the onions, celery, and carrots into the pot and cook until the veggies begin to soften (5-8 min.).
3.   Pour in the chicken stock, bay leaf, salt, pepper, and thyme.
4.   Once boiling, lower the heat setting to simmer. Add the whole chicken breast. Place a top on the soup pot and simmer for an additional 15-20 minutes.
5.   Take the pan from the heat. Trash the bay leaf. Carefully take

the chicken from the pot. Place on a cutting surface to shred.

6. Toss the shredded chicken back into the pot and simmer until it's done (5 min.).
7. Pour in the milk and parsley, cooking until hot and serve.

Creamy Asparagus Soup

Yields Provided: 2 Servings
Nutritional Counts Per Serving:
- **Calories:** 157
- **Net Carbs:** 3 g
- **Total Fat Content:** 13 g
- **Protein:** 7 g

Ingredients Needed:
- Asparagus with juices (15 oz. can)
- Chicken broth (1.5 cups)
- Onion powder (.5 tsp.)
- Marjoram (.25 tsp.)
- Black pepper (.25 tsp.)
- Garlic powder (.25 tsp.)
- Heavy cream (.25 cup)
- Salt (as desired)
- Fresh parsley (1 tbsp.)

How to Prepare:
1. Remove the asparagus from the can. Add enough broth to fill the asparagus can.
2. Roughly chop the asparagus and add the juices into a medium pot. Puree using an immersion blender until creamy. Stir in the seasonings and reduce the heat. Add the parsley and simmer until hot.
3. Season with salt if desired and serve.

Crockpot Chicken Chowder

Yields Provided: 4 Servings
Nutritional Counts Per Serving:
- **Calories**: 457
- **Net Carbs**: 7.5 g
- **Total Fat Content**: 29 g
- **Protein**: 40 g

Ingredients Needed:
- Garlic clove (1)
- Cilantro (1 tbsp.)
- Small onion (1)
- Cream cheese (8 oz.)
- Chicken broth (1 cup)
- Chicken breasts – skinless & boneless (1 lb.)
- Diced tomatoes (14 oz.)
- Diced jalapeño (.5 oz.)
- Freshly squeezed lime juice (1.6 oz)
- Black pepper (1 tbsp.)
- Salt (1 tsp.)

How to Prepare:
1. Chop the garlic and cilantro. Dice the onion and jalapeño.
2. Combine all of the fixings in the crockpot. Prepare on the low-temperature setting for 6-9 hours or high for four hours.
3. Once it is done, shred the chicken in the pot using two forks.
4. Serve.

Egg Drop Soup

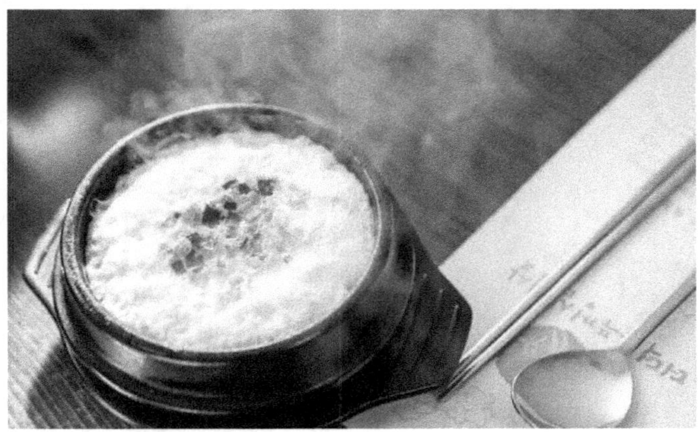

Yields Provided: 6 Servings

Nutritional Counts Per Serving:

- **Calories**: 255
- **Net Carbs**: 3 g
- **Total Fat Content**: 22 g
- **Protein**: 11 g

Ingredients Needed:

- Vegetable broth (2 quarts)
- Minced garlic cloves (2)
- Freshly chopped ginger (1 tbsp.)
- Turmeric (1 tbsp.)
- Sliced chili pepper (1 small)
- Coconut aminos (2 tbsp.)
- Large eggs (4)
- Mushrooms (2 cups sliced)
- Chopped spinach (4 cups)
- Sliced spring onions (2 medium)
- Freshly chopped cilantro (2 tbsp.)
- Black pepper (to your liking)
- Pink Himalayan (1 tsp.)
- Olive oil for serving (6 tbsp.)

How to Prepare:
1. Grate the ginger root and turmeric. Mince the garlic cloves and slice the peppers and mushrooms.
2. Chop the chard stalks and leaves. Separate the stalks from the leaves.
3. Dump the vegetable stock into a soup pot and simmer until it begins to boil. Toss in the garlic, ginger, turmeric, chard stalks, mushrooms, coconut aminos, and chili peppers. Boil for approximately five minutes.
4. Fold in the chard leaves and simmer for one minute.
5. Whip the eggs in a dish and add them slowly to the soup mixture. Stir until the egg is done and set it on the countertop.
6. Slice the onions and chop the cilantro. Toss them into the pot.
7. Pour into serving bowls and drizzle with some olive oil (1 tbsp. per serving).
8. Serve warm or chilled.

Greens Soup

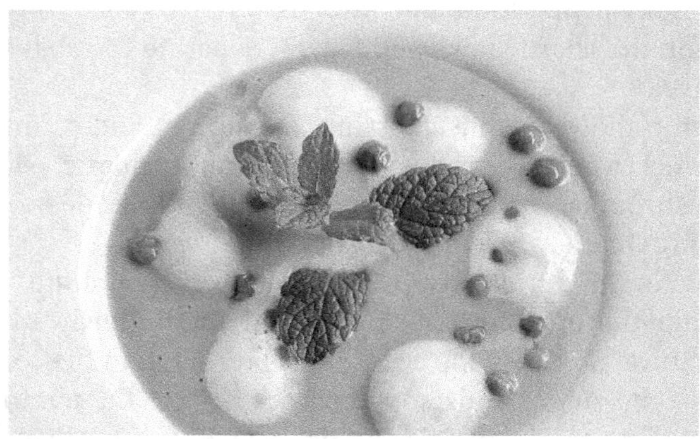

Yields Provided: 6 Servings
Nutritional Counts Per Serving:
- **Calories**: 191
- **Net Carbs**: 6 g
- **Total Fat Content**: 8 g
- **Protein**: 6.3 g

Ingredients Needed:
- Spinach leaves (2 cups)
- Diced avocado (1)
- Diced English cucumber (.5 cup)
- Gluten-free vegetable broth (.25 cup)
- Black pepper and salt (as desired)

How to Prepare:
1. Combine each of the fixings in the blender.
2. Toss in the fresh herbs and serve.

Shirataki Soup

Yields Provided: 2 Servings
Nutritional Counts Per Serving:
- **Calories**: 130
- **Protein**: 1 g
- **Net Carbs**: 1.5 g
- **Total Fat Content**: 12 g

Ingredients Needed:
- Chicken stock (3 cups)
- Minced ginger (1 tsp.)
- Cardamom (.25 tsp.)
- Minced garlic clove (1)
- Mushrooms – your choice (.5 cup)
- *Optional*: Chili sauce (1 tsp.)
- Chopped cilantro (to taste)
- Thinly sliced chili pepper (1)
- Boneless - skinless chicken thighs (2)

How to Prepare:
1. On the stovetop, use the med-high heat setting to warm the stock.
2. Toss in the ginger, garlic, mushrooms, and cardamom. Simmer for about ten minutes.
3. Fold in the chicken. Cook for about five minutes.
4. Prepare two soup dishes and add the sliced chili pepper to each dish.
5. Serve the soup and garnish with the cilantro and spices you like.

Spring Soup with Poached Egg

Yields Provided: 2 Servings
Nutritional Counts Per Serving:
- **Calories:** 150
- **Net Carbs:** 4 g
- **Total Fat Content:** 5 g
- **Protein:** 16 g

Ingredients Needed:
- Eggs (2)
- Chicken broth (1 qt. - 32 oz.)
- Chopped romaine lettuce (1 head)
  Salt (as desired)

How to Prepare:
1. Bring a pan of the chicken broth to a boil.
2. For a slightly runny egg, turn down the heat, and poach the two eggs in the broth for five minutes.
3. Remove the eggs and set aside into two serving dishes for now.
4. Chop the lettuce and toss into the broth. Simmer for a few minutes until slightly wilted.
5. Ladle the broth with the lettuce into the bowls with eggs and serve.

Chapter 4: Dinner: Poultry Options

BBQ Chicken Zucchini Boats

Yields Provided: 4 Servings
Nutritional Counts Per Serving:
- **Calories**: 212
- **Net Carbs**: 9 g
- **Total Fat Content**: 11 g
- **Protein**: 19 g

Ingredients Needed:
- Zucchini (3 halved)
- Chicken breast (1 lb. cooked)
- BBQ sauce (.5 cup)
- Shredded Mexican cheese (.33 cup)
- Avocado (1 sliced)
- Halved cherry tomatoes (.5 cup)
- Diced green onions (.25 cup)
- Keto-friendly ranch dressing (3 tbsp.)
- *Also Needed:* 9x13 casserole dish

How to Prepare:
1. Set the oven to reach 350° Fahrenheit.
2. Use a sharp knife and cut the zucchini in half. Discard the seeds. Make the boat by carving out of the center. Place the zucchini flesh side up into the casserole dish.
3. Discard and cut the skin and bones from the chicken. Shred and add the chicken in with the barbeque sauce. Toss to coat all the chicken fully.
4. Fill the zucchini boats with the mixture using about .25 to .33 cup each.
5. Sprinkle with Mexican cheese on top.
6. Bake for approximately 15 minutes. (If you would like it tenderer; bake for an additional 5 to 10 minutes to reach the

desired tenderness.)

7. Remove from the oven. Top it off with avocado, green onion, tomatoes, and a drizzle of dressing. Serve.

Cashew Chicken Curry

Yields Provided: 4 Servings
Nutritional Counts Per Serving:
- **Calories**: 364
- **Net Carbs**: 14 g
- **Total Fat Content**: 18 g
- **Protein**: 34 g

Ingredients Needed:
- Cauliflower (4 cups)
- Fresh tomatoes (2 large)
- Red onion (1 medium)
- Cucumber (2 cups)
- Coconut oil (2 tbsp.)
- Yellow curry powder - divided (1 tbsp. (+) .5 tsp.)
- Sea salt & Black pepper (as desired)
- Roasted - salted cashews (.66 cup)
- Breasts of chicken (4 small - 1 lb.)
- Egg white (1 large)
- *For the Garnish:*
- Freshly chopped fresh mint
- Minced fresh cilantro
- *Also Needed:* Food processor & Rimmed baking sheet

How to Prepare:
1. Chop the cauliflower into florets and quarter the tomatoes. Roughly chop the onion and thinly slice the cucumber into halves. Remove the skin and bones from the chicken.
2. Heat the oven to 425° Fahrenheit.
3. Toss the quartered tomatoes, cauliflower florets, and onion into a mixing container. Melt the coconut oil and sprinkle

using 1.5 teaspoons of curry powder. Mix until well.

4. Arrange on a baking sheet in one layer. Dust with pepper and salt to your liking. Add the rest of the curry powder and cashews into a food processor. Pulse leaving a few chunks for texture.
5. Pat to remove the moisture from the chicken breasts using a paper towel.
6. Put the egg white and cashews into two shallow plates.
7. Dredge the chicken through the egg white. Shake off any excess, and press into the cashews.
8. Flip and lightly press the other side into the cashews.
9. Put the chicken breast onto a small cooling rack that fits on your sheet pan (one with legs is preferred so it sits over the veggies).
10. Continue the process with the remainder of the chicken. Place the cooling rack over a sheet pan (over the top of the veggies).
11. Bake the chicken to reach an internal temperature of 165° Fahrenheit (14-15 min.). Once it's done, toss the fresh cucumbers onto the pan. Garnish with mint and cilantro.

Chicken Asparagus Dinner

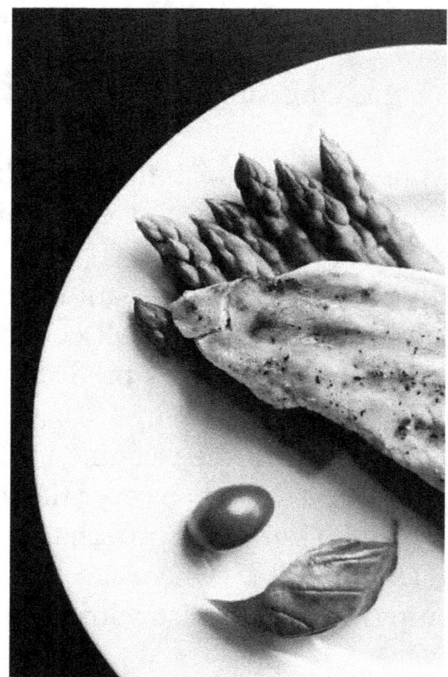

Yields Provided: 8 Servings
Nutritional Counts Per Serving:
- **Calories**: 439
- **Net Carbs**: 4 g
- **Total Fat Content**: 18 g
- **Protein**: 63 g

Ingredients Needed:
- Chicken breasts (4 lb.)
- Sun-dried tomatoes (4)
- Thick-cut bacon (4 slices)
- Avocado oil (1 tbsp.)
- Trimmed asparagus (1 lb.)
- Salt (1 tsp.)
- Pepper (.25 tsp.)
- Provolone cheese (8 slices)
- *Also Needed*: 1 baking pan

How to Prepare:

1. Set the oven temperature to 400° Fahrenheit.
2. Cut the chicken breasts into eight thin pieces. Chop the bacon and tomatoes into one-inch pieces.
3. Pour the oil into the baking pan along with the chicken and asparagus. Top it off with the tomatoes and bacon.
4. Sprinkle some pepper and salt for seasoning.
5. Bake until the chicken reaches 160° Fahrenheit (internally) or about 25 minutes.
6. Toss in the asparagus and cheese.
7. Garnish with a portion of bacon and tomatoes.
8. Bake for another three to four minutes until the cheese has melted.

Chicken Nuggets

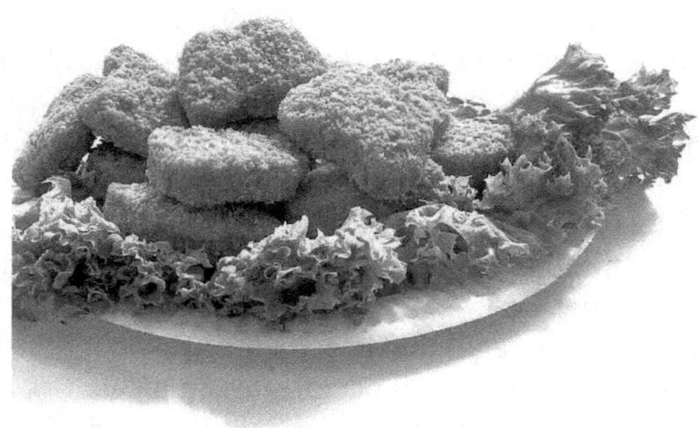

Yields Provided: 6 Servings
Nutritional Counts Per Serving:
- **Calories**: 243
- **Net Carbs**: 2 g
- **Total Fat Content**: 17 g
- **Protein**: 18 g

Ingredients Needed:
- Egg (1)
- Cooked chicken (2 cups)
- Cream cheese (8 oz.)
- Almond flour (.25 cup)
- Garlic salt (1 tsp.)

How to Prepare:
1. Warm the oven to reach 350º Fahrenheit.
2. Lightly spritz a baking pan using cooking oil spray or layer it with a sheet of parchment baking paper.
3. Shred the chicken using a food processor. Try using a combination of white and dark meat - your choice.
4. Stir in the rest of the fixings and combine well.
5. Drop the nugget mixture onto the prepared baking tin. Bake

until firm and slightly browned (12-14 min.).

Creamy Chicken & Greens

Yields Provided: 4 Servings
Nutritional Counts Per Serving:
- **Calories**: 446
- **Net Carbs**: 3 g
- **Total Fat Content**: 38 g
- **Protein**: 18 g

Ingredients Needed:
- Chicken thighs – skins on (1 lb.)
- Chicken stock (1 cup)
- Cream (1 cup)
- Coconut oil (2 tbsp.)
- Italian herbs (1 tsp.)
- Dark leafy greens (2 cups)
- Pepper & Salt (your preference)
- Coconut flour (2 tbsp.)
- Melted butter (2 tbsp.)

How to Prepare:
1. On the stovetop, add oil in a skillet using the med-high temperature setting.
2. Remove the bones from the chicken and dust using salt and pepper. Fry the chicken until done.
3. Make the sauce by adding the butter to a saucepan. Whisk in the flour to form a thick paste. Slowly, whisk in the cream. Once it boils, mix in the herbs.
4. Transfer the chicken to the counter and add the stock. Deglaze the pan, and whisk the cream sauce. Toss in the greens until thoroughly coated with the sauce.
5. Arrange the thighs on the greens, warm up, and serve.

**Curry Chicken Lettuce Wraps**

Yields Provided: 5 Servings
Nutritional Counts Per Serving:
- **Calories**: 554
- **Net Carbs**: 7 g
- **Total Fat Content**: 36 g
- **Protein**: 50 g

Ingredients Needed:
Minced garlic cloves (2)
Minced onion (.25 cup)
Chicken thighs – skinless & boneless (1 lb.)
Ghee (3 tbsp.)
Black pepper (1 tsp.)
Curry powder (2 tsp.)
Salt (1.5 tsp.)
Riced cauliflower (1 cup)
Lettuce leaves (5-6)
Keto-friendly sour cream (as desired - count the carbs)

How to Prepare:
1. Mince the garlic and onions. Set aside for now.
2. Discard the bones and skin from the chicken and dice into one-inch pieces.
3. On the stovetop, add 2 tbsp. of ghee to a skillet and melt. Toss in the onion and sauté until browned. Fold in the chicken and sprinkle with the garlic, pepper, and salt.
4. Cook for eight minutes. Stir in the remainder of the ghee, riced cauliflower, and curry. Stir until well mixed.
5. Prepare the lettuce leaves and add the mixture.
6. Serve with a dollop of cream.

Fettuccine Chicken Alfredo

Yields Provided: 2 Servings
Nutritional Counts Per Serving:
- **Calories:** 585
- **Net Carbs:** 1 g
- **Total Fat Content:** 51 g
- **Protein:** 25 g

Ingredients Needed:
- Butter (2 tbsp.)
- Minced garlic cloves (2)
- Dried basil (.5 tsp.)
- Heavy cream (.5 cup)
- Grated parmesan (4 tbsp.)

Ingredients Needed - For the Chicken & Noodles
- Chicken thighs - no bones or skin (2)
- Olive oil (1 tbsp.)
- Miracle Noodle - Fettuccini (1 bag)
- Black pepper & salt (as desired)

How to Prepare:
1. *For the Sauce:* Measure and toss the butter and cloves into a pan. Sauté for two minutes. Pour the cream into the skillet and simmer two additional minutes.
2. Toss in one tablespoon of the parmesan at a time. Add the pepper, salt, and dried basil. Simmer 3 to 5 minutes on the low-heat temperature setting.
3. *For the Chicken:* Pound the chicken with a meat tenderizer hammer until it's ½-inch thick. Warm up the oil in a frying pan using the medium heat setting. Toss in the chicken to simmer for approximately seven minutes per side. Shred and set aside.
4. *For the Noodles:* Prepare the package of noodles. Boil them for

two minutes in a pot of water.

5. Fold in the noodles along with the sauce and shredded chicken. Cook slowly for two minutes and serve.

Nacho Chicken Casserole

Yields Provided: 6 Servings
Nutritional Counts Per Serving:
- **Calories**: 426
- **Net Carbs**: 4.3 g
- **Total Fat Content**: 32.2 g
- **Protein**: 31 g

Ingredients Needed:
- Jalapeño pepper (1 medium)
- Chicken thighs (1.75 lb.)
- Pepper and salt (to taste)
- Olive oil (2 tbsp.)
- Chili seasoning (1.5 tsp.)
- Cheddar cheese (4 oz.)
- Cream cheese (4 oz.)
- Parmesan cheese (3 tbsp.)
- Green chilies and tomatoes (1 cup)
- Sour cream (.25 cup)
- Frozen cauliflower (1 pkg.)
- *Also Needed:* Immersion blender

How to Prepare:
1. Warm the oven to reach 375º Fahrenheit.
2. Slice the jalapeño into pieces and set aside.
3. Cutaway the skin and bones from the chicken. Chop it and sprinkle using the pepper and salt. Prepare in a skillet using a portion of olive oil on the med-high temperature setting until browned.
4. Blend in the sour cream, cream cheese, and ¾ of the cheddar cheese. Stir until melted and combined well. Pour in the tomatoes and chilies. Stir and add it all to a baking dish.
5. Cook the cauliflower in the microwave. Blend in the rest of the cheese with the immersion blender until it resembles mashed

potatoes. Season as desired.

6. Spread the cauliflower concoction over the casserole and sprinkle with the peppers. Bake approximately 15 to 20 minutes.

Pesto & Mozzarella Chicken Casserole

Yields Provided: 8 Servings
Nutritional Counts Per Serving:
- **Calories**: 451
- **Net Carbs**: 3 g
- **Total Fat Content**: 30 g
- **Protein**: 38 g

Ingredients Needed:
- Cooking oil (as needed)
- Grilled & cubed chicken breasts (2 lb.)
- Cubed mozzarella (8 oz.)
- Cream cheese (8 oz.)
- Shredded mozzarella (8 oz.)
- Pesto (.25 cup)
- Heavy cream (.25 to .5 cup)

How to Prepare:
1. Warm the oven to 400° Fahrenheit. Spritz a casserole dish with a spritz of cooking oil spray.
2. Combine the pesto, heavy cream, and softened cream cheese.
3. Add the chicken and cubed mozzarella into the greased dish.
4. Sprinkle the chicken using the shredded mozzarella. Bake for 25-30 minutes.
5. *Tip*: Use 1/2 cup of cream if you prefer a thinner sauce or 1/4 cup for a thicker choice.

Rotisserie Chicken & Cabbage Shreds

Yields Provided: 2 Servings
Nutritional Counts Per Serving:
- **Calories:** 423
- **Net Carbs:** 6 g
- **Total Fat Content:** 35 g
- **Protein:** 17 g

Ingredients Needed:
- Red onion (.5 of 1)
- Fresh green cabbage (7 oz.)
- Precooked rotisserie chicken (1 lb.)
- Keto-friendly mayo (.5 cup)
- Olive oil (1 tbsp.)
- Pepper & Salt (to your liking)

How to Prepare:
1. Use a sharp kitchen knife to shred the cabbage and slice the onion into thin slices.
2. Place the chicken on a platter, add the mayo, and a drizzle of oil. Dust using salt and pepper. Serve.

Slow-Cooked Teriyaki

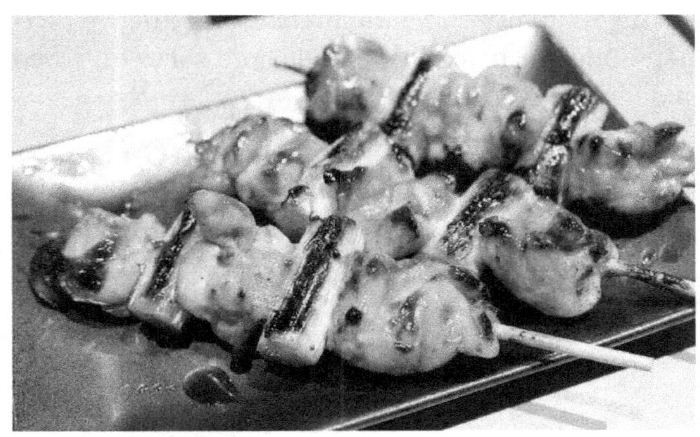

Yields Provided: 6 Servings
Nutritional Counts Per Serving:

- **Calories**: 158
- **Net Carbs**: 4 g
- **Total Fat Content**: 6 g
- **Protein**: 20 g

Ingredients Needed:

Red pepper (2)
Yellow onion (1)
Garlic cloves (3)
Reduced-sodium beef broth (.5 cup)
Coconut aminos (.25 cup)
Water (.33 cup)
Knob freshly grated ginger (1-inch piece)
Pepper & salt (as desired)
Chicken thighs (2 lb.)
For the Garnish: 4 green onions
Optional for Serving: Lettuce leaves

How to Prepare:

Chop the peppers, onions, and garlic.

Whisk the water, aminos, and broth – adding it to the cooker.
Blend in the rest of the fixings (omitting the lettuce and green onions).
Cook for six hours using the high heat setting.
When done; garnish with onions, and serve on a bed of lettuce as a delicious taco.

Chapter 5: Dinner: Seafood Selections

Avocado & Salmon Omelet Wrap

Yields Provided: 2 Servings
Nutritional Counts Per Serving:
- **Calories**: 765
- **Net Carbs**: 6 g
- **Total Fat Content**: 67 g
- **Protein**: 37 g

Ingredients Needed:
- Large eggs (3)
- Smoked salmon (1.8 oz.)
- Avocado (.5 of 1 average-size)
- Spring onion (1)
- Cream cheese - full-fat (2 tbsp)
- Chives - freshly chopped (2 tbsp.)
- Butter or ghee (1 tbsp.)
- Pepper and salt (as desired)

How to Prepare:
1. Add a sprinkle of pepper and salt to the eggs. Use a fork or whisk—mixing them well. Blend in the chives and cream cheese.
2. Prepare the salmon and avocado (peel and slice or chop).
3. Combine the butter/ghee and the egg mixture in a frying pan. Continue cooking on low heat until done.
4. Place the omelet on a serving dish with a portion of cheese over it. Sprinkle the onion, prepared avocado, and salmon into the wrap.
5. Close and serve!

Baked Tilapia with Cherry Tomatoes

Yields Provided: 2 Servings
Nutritional Counts Per Serving:
- **Calories**: 180
- **Net Carbs**: 4 g
- **Total Fat Content**: 8 g
- **Protein**: 23 g

Ingredients Needed:
- Butter (2 tsp.)
- Tilapia fillets (2 - 4 oz. each)
- Cherry tomatoes (8)
- Pitted black olives (.25 cup)
- Salt (.5 tsp.)
- Paprika (.25 tsp.)
- Black pepper (.25 tsp.)
- Garlic powder (1 tsp.)
- Freshly squeezed lemon juice (1 tbsp.)
- *Optional*: Balsamic vinegar (1 tbsp.)

How to Prepare:
1. Warm the oven to reach 375° Fahrenheit.
2. Grease a roasting pan and add the butter along with the olives and tomatoes.
3. Season the tilapia with the spices. Lastly, add the fish fillets into the pan with a spritz of the lemon juice.
4. Add a piece of foil over the pan. Bake until the fish easily flakes (25 to 30 min.).
5. Garnish with the vinegar if desired.

Beetroot-Cured Salmon with Dill Oil

Yields Provided: 4 Servings
Nutritional Counts Per Serving:
- **Calories:** 500
- **Net Carbs:** 4 g
- **Total Fat Content:** 42 g
- **Protein:** 25 g

Ingredients Needed:
- Beet (1)
- Salt (2 tbsp.)
- White peppercorns (5)
- Lime - zested (1)
- Salmon (1 lb.)

Ingredients Needed - Dill Oil:
- Chopped fresh dill (.5 cup)
- Frozen spinach (1 tbsp.)
- Light olive oil or avocado oil (.5 cup)
- Salt and pepper (to your liking)

Ingredients Needed - Serving:
- Daikon - finely sliced (2 oz.)
- Lettuce (.5 lb.)

How to Prepare:
1. Rinse the beetroot thoroughly and peel. Grate it coarsely and add it to a bowl along with the salt, peppercorn, and lime zest.
2. Partially defrost the salmon before the curing process.
3. Arrange the salmon with the skin side down and rub the flesh side evenly through the beetroot mixture. (You should probably wear a pair of gloves on your hands to prevent staining.)
4. Arrange the salmon in a glass dish with a piece of film over the top. Marinate in the fridge for one to two days, flipping halfway through the process.

5. Combine the spinach and dill with a hand blender. Mix in the oil, salt, and pepper.
6. Unwrap the salmon and brush off the beetroot cure (don't serve the marinade).
7. Cut the fish into thin slices and serve with a portion of dill oil, chopped bacon, and leafy greens.

Chipotle Fish Tacos

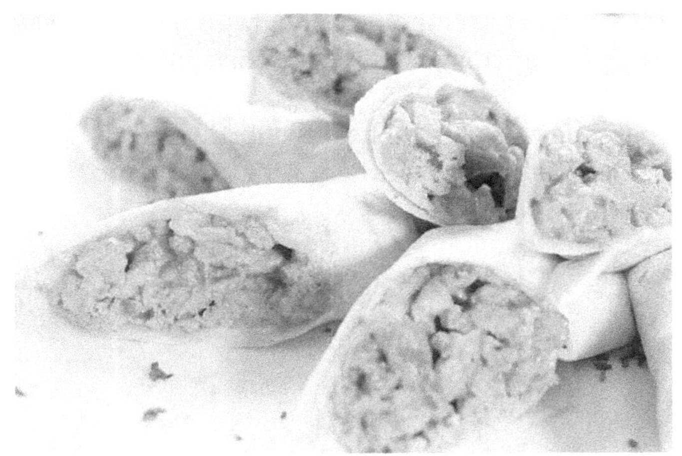

Yields Provided: 4 Servings
Nutritional Counts Per Serving:
- **Calories**: 300
- **Net Carbs**: 7 g
- **Total Fat Content**: 20 g
- **Protein**: 24 g

Ingredients Needed:
- Jalapeño (1)
- Small yellow onion (.5 of 1)
- Pressed garlic (2 cloves)
- Chipotle peppers in adobo sauce (4 oz.)
- Olive oil (2 tbsp.)
- Mayonnaise (2 tbsp.)
- Butter (2 tbsp.)
- Low-carb tortillas (4)
- Haddock fillets (1 lb. - 4 fillets)

How to Prepare:
1. Dice the onion and chop the jalapeño.
2. In a skillet, fry the onion for about five minutes using the med-

high heat setting.

3. Lower the heat setting to medium. Toss in the garlic and jalapeño. Stir for another 2 minutes.
4. Chop and add the chipotles, along with the adobo sauce.
5. Toss in butter, mayonnaise, and fish into the pan. Fry for 8 minutes.
6. Prepare the tacos. Fry to heat the tortilla for about two minutes per side. Chill and shape them with the fish mixture.

Cod - Skillet Fried

Yields Provided: 4 Servings
Nutritional Counts Per Serving:
- **Calories**: 160
- **Net Carbs**: 1 g
- **Total Fat Content**: 7 g
- **Protein**: 21 g

Ingredients Needed:
- Ghee (3 tbsp.)
- Minced garlic cloves (6)
- Cod fillets (4 @.33 lb. ea.)
- *Optional:* Garlic powder
- *Optional:* Salt

How to Prepare:
1. Melt the ghee and add half of the garlic into a skillet.
2. Arrange the fillets in the pan using med-high heat. Sprinkle with the garlic, pepper, and salt.
3. Once it turns white halfway up its side, turn it over, and add the remainder of the minced garlic. Continue cooking until it flakes easily.
4. Serve with a portion of ghee or garlic from the pan.

Fish Cakes

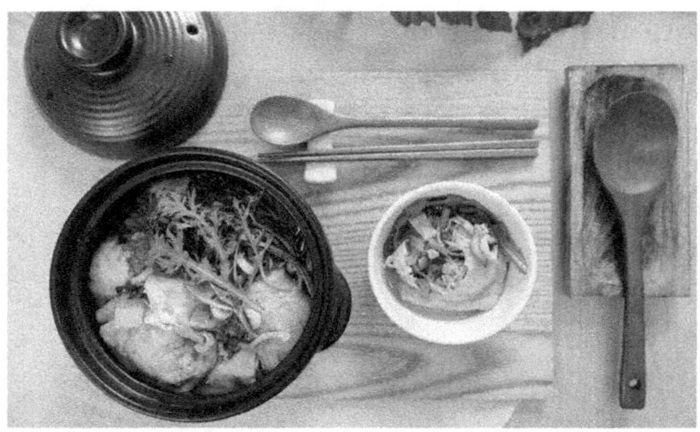

Yields Provided: 6 Servings

Nutritional Counts Per Serving:
- **Net Carbs**: 0.6 g
- **Calories**: 69
- **Total Fat Content**: 6.5 g
- **Protein**: 1.1 g

Ingredients Needed:
- Wild-caught raw white boneless fish (1 lb.)
- Cilantro - leaves and stems (.25 cup)
- Pinch of salt (1 pinch)
- Chili flakes (1 pinch)
- Coconut oil/ ghee - for frying (1-2 tbsp.)
- Avocado or a neutral oil - for greasing your hands (as needed)
- Avocados (2 ripe)
- Lemon (1 juiced)
- Salt (1 pinch)
- Water (2 tbsp.)
- *Optional*: Garlic cloves (1-2)
- *Also Needed*: Blender or food processor

How to Prepare:
1. Toss the fish, herbs, garlic, salt, chili, and fish into a food processor. Blitz until everything is combined evenly.

2. Using the med-high heat setting; add the ghee or coconut oil into a large skillet. Swirl the pan to coat.
3. Oil your hands and roll the fish mixture into 6 patties.
4. Add the cakes to the heated frying pan. Simmer until golden brown.
5. While the fish cakes are cooking, add all of the dipping sauce fixings (starting with the lemon juice) into a blender. Blitz until creamy. Taste the mixture and add more lemon juice or salt if desired.
6. When the fish cakes are cooked, serve warm with dipping sauce.

Garlic & Lemon Shrimp Pasta

Yields Provided: 4 Servings
Nutritional Counts Per Serving:
- **Calories**: 360
- **Net Carbs**: 3.5 g
- **Total Fat Content**: 21 g
- **Protein**: 36 g

Ingredients Needed:
- Miracle Noodle Angel Hair Pasta (2 pkg.)
- Garlic cloves (4)
- Olive oil (2 tbsp.)
- Butter (2 tbsp.)
- Large raw shrimp (1 lb.)
- Lemon (.5 of 1)
- Paprika (.5 tsp.)
- Fresh basil (as desired)
- Pepper and salt (to taste)

How to Prepare:
1. Drain the water from the package of noodles and rinse them in cold water. Toss into a pot of boiling water for two minutes. Transfer to a hot skillet over medium heat to remove the excess liquid (dry roast). Set them aside.
2. Use the same pan to warm the butter, oil, and mashed garlic. Sauté for a few minutes but _don't_ brown.
3. Slice the lemon into rounds and add them to the garlic along with the shrimp. Sauté for approximately three minutes on each side.
4. Fold in the noodles and spices and stir to blend the flavors.

Sesame Ginger Salmon

Yields Provided: 2 Servings
Nutritional Counts Per Serving:
- **Calories**: 370
- **Net Carbs**: 2.5 g
- **Total Fat Content**: 24 g
- **Protein**: 33 g

Ingredients Needed:
- Salmon fillet (1 - 10 oz.)
- Minced ginger (1-2 tsp.)
- White wine (2 tbsp.)
- Sesame oil (2 tsp.)
- Rice vinegar (1 tbsp.)
- Keto-friendly soy sauce substitute (2 tbsp.)
- Sugar-free ketchup (1 tbsp.)
- Fish sauce – Red Boat (1 tbsp.)

How to Prepare:
1. Combine all of the fixings in a plastic canister with a tight-fitting lid (omit the ketchup, oil, and wine for now). Marinade them for about 10 to 15 minutes.
2. On the stovetop, prepare a skillet using the high-heat temperature setting. Pour in the oil. Add the fish when it's hot, skin side down.
3. Brown both sides for three to four minutes.
4. Pour in the marinated juices to the pan to simmer when the fish is flipped. Arrange the fish on two dinner plates.
5. Pour in the wine and ketchup to the pan and simmer five minutes until it's reduced. Serve with your favorite vegetable.

<u>*Shrimp Alfredo*</u>

Yields Provided: 4 Servings
Nutritional Counts Per Serving:
- **Calories**: 298
- **Net Carbs**: 6.5 g
- **Total Fat Content**: 18 g
- **Protein**: 23 g

Ingredients Needed:
- Raw shrimp (1 lb.)
- Salted butter (1 tbsp.)
- Cubed cream cheese (4 oz.)
- Whole milk (.5 cup)
- Garlic powder (1 tbsp.)
- Shredded parmesan cheese (.5 cup)
- Salt (1 tsp.)
- Dried basil (1 tsp.)
- Baby kale or spinach (.25 cup)
- Whole sun-dried tomatoes (5)
- *Also Needed:* Food processor or blender

How to Prepare:
1. Heat up the butter using the medium heat setting in a skillet.
2. Toss in the shrimp and lower the heat to med-low.
3. After 30 seconds, flip the shrimp and cook until slightly pink. Blend in the cream cheese.
4. Increase the heat and pour in the milk. Stir frequently.
5. Sprinkle with the salt, basil, and garlic. Empty the parmesan cheese in, and mix well.
6. Simmer until the sauce has thickened. Cut the sun-dried tomatoes into strips.
7. Lastly, fold in the kale/spinach and dried tomatoes. Serve steaming hot.

Tangy Shrimp

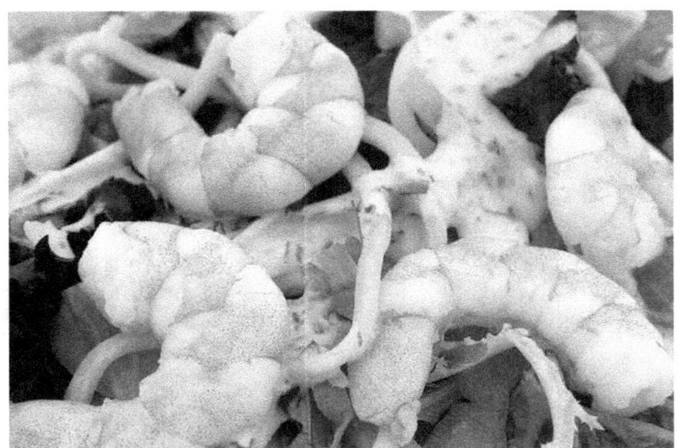

Yields Provided: 2 Servings

Nutritional Counts Per Serving:

- **Calories**: 335
- **Net Carbs**: 3 g
- **Total Fat Content**: 27 g
- **Protein**: 23 g

Ingredients Needed:

- Garlic (3 cloves)
- Olive oil (.25 cup)
- Large shrimp (.5 lb.)
- Lemon (1 - cut into wedges)
- Cayenne pepper (to your liking)
- Pepper and salt (to your liking)

How to Prepare:

1. Sauté the garlic and cayenne along with the olive oil using the medium heat temperature setting.
2. Peel and devein the shrimp. Cook 2 to 3 minutes on each side.
3. Season using pepper, salt, and lemon wedges.
4. Use the rest of the garlic oil for a dipping sauce.

Bacon Cheeseburger

Yields Provided: 12 Servings - 2 each
Nutritional Counts Per Serving:
- **Calories**: 489
- **Net Carbs**: 0.8 g
- **Total Fat Content**: 41 g
- **Protein**: 27 g

Ingredients Needed:
- Low-sodium bacon (16 oz. pkg.)
- Ground beef (3 lb.)
- Shredded cheddar cheese (8 oz.)
- Eggs (2)
- Medium chopped onion (.5 of 1)

How to Prepare:
1. Fry the bacon and chop to bits. Shred the cheese and dice the onion.
2. Combine the mixture with the beef and blend in the whipped eggs.
3. Prepare 24 burgers and grill them the way you like them.

BBQ Flank Steak

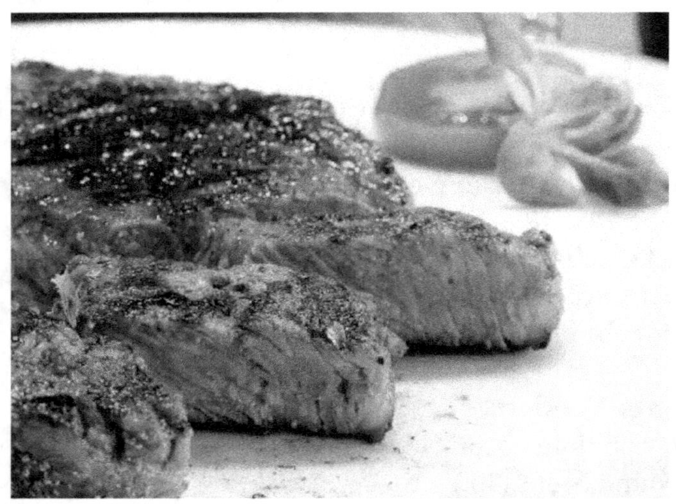

Yields Provided: 8 Servings
Nutritional Counts Per Serving:
- **Calories**: 342
- **Net Carbs**: 1 g
- **Total Fat Content**: 21 g
- **Protein**: 35 g

Ingredients Needed:
- Coconut aminos (1 tbsp.)
- Melted butter (2 tbsp.)
- Flank steak (3 lb.)
- Granulated garlic (1 tsp.)
- Paprika (1 tsp.)
- Cayenne pepper (1 tsp.)
- Granulated onion (1 tsp.)
- White pepper (1 tsp.)
- Salt (1 tsp.)
- Black pepper (1 tsp.)
- Water (.25 cup)
- *Also Needed:* Slow Cooker

How to Prepare:
1. Combine the aminos, seasonings, and melted butter. Rub into the steak.
2. Add the water to the cooker and the steak fixings.
3. Cook for 8 hours (flipping halfway through the cooking cycle).
4. Serve.

___Cheeseburger Calzone___

Yields Provided: 8 Servings
Nutritional Counts Per Serving:
- **Calories:** 580
- **Net Carbs:** 3 g
- **Total Fat Content:** 47 g
- **Protein:** 34 g

Ingredients Needed:
- Dill pickle spears (4)
- Cream cheese – divided (8 oz.)
- Shredded mozzarella cheese (1 cup)
- Egg (1)
- Yellow diced onion (.5 of 1)
- Ground beef - lean (1.5 lb.)
- Thick-cut bacon strips (4)
- Almond flour (1 cup)
- Mayonnaise (.5 cup)
- Shredded cheddar cheese (1 cup)

How to Prepare:
1. Program the oven temperature setting to 425° Fahrenheit. Prepare a cookie tin with parchment paper.
2. Chop the pickles into spears. Set aside for now.
3. Prepare the crust. Combine half of the cream cheese and mozzarella cheese. Microwave 35 seconds. When it melts, add the egg and almond flour to make the dough. Set aside.
4. Cook the beef on the stovetop using the medium heat setting.
5. Prepare the bacon until crunchy (microwave for five minutes or stovetop). When cool, break into bits.
6. Dice the onion and add to the beef. Cook until softened. Toss in the bacon, cheddar cheese, pickle bits, the rest of the cream cheese, and mayonnaise. Stir well.
7. Roll the dough onto the prepared baking tin. Scoop the mixture into the center. Fold the ends and side to make the calzone.

8. Bake until browned or about 15 minutes. Let it rest for 10 minutes before slicing.

Feta-Stuffed Burgers

Yields Provided: 2 Servings
Nutritional Counts Per Serving:
- **Calories**: 607
- **Net Carbs**: 1 g
- **Total Fat Content**: 48 g
- **Protein**: 41 g

Ingredients Needed:
- Scallion (1)
- Ground beef and lamb (12 oz. total – 6 oz. each)
- Chopped mint leaves (2 tbsp.)
- Ghee (1 tbsp.)
- Dijon mustard (1 tbsp.)
- Crumbled feta cheese (2 oz.)
- Pink salt and Black pepper (to your liking)

How to Prepare:
1. Thinly slice the green and white parts of the scallion. Also, finely chop the fresh mint leaves. Crumble the feta.
2. Combine the mustard with the mint and scallions. Stir in the beef and lamb. Mix well and shape into four patties. Sprinkle with salt and pepper.
3. Press the feta cubes into two of the patties and place a patty on top (cheese in the middle). Seal it closed.
4. Using the medium heat setting, melt the ghee and add the patties once the pan is hot. Cook each side for 5 minutes and serve.

Ground Beef Veggie Skillet

Yields Provided: 4 Servings
Nutritional Counts Per Serving:
- **Calories**: 261
- **Net Carbs**: 6 g
- **Total Fat Content**: 13 g
- **Protein**: 30 g

Ingredients Needed:
- Clove of garlic (1)
- Onions (.5 cup)
- Red bell peppers (.5 cup)
- Zucchini (1 medium)
- Asparagus (.5 lb.)
- Extra-virgin olive oil (2 tbsp.)
- Extra-lean ground beef (1 lb.)
- Dijon mustard (1 tsp.)
- Tomato passata or tomato sauce (.25 cup)
- Dried oregano (.5 tsp.)
- *Optional*: Crushed red pepper (.125 tsp.)
- Black pepper & salt (as desired)
- *Toppings*:
- Crumbled feta cheese (1 tbsp.)
- Freshly chopped parsley (as desired)

How to Prepare:
1. Mince or dice the garlic, onions, and peppers. Quarter the zucchini and slice the asparagus into three segments each.
2. Heat a large skillet using the med-high heat setting, and pour in the olive oil.
3. Toss in the garlic and beef. Break apart as it is cooking. Stir occasionally, and cook for about seven minutes until it's no longer pink. Transfer the meat from the skillet, and set aside for now.
4. Fold in the onions and red bell peppers, and simmer until the

onions are softened or about three to four minutes. Pour in a little bit of olive oil to sauté the veggies - as needed.
5. Toss in the zucchini and asparagus. Simmer for another three to five minutes.
6. Return the beef to the skillet, and mix everything together.
7. Simmer for one to two additional minutes.
8. Garnish with fresh parsley and feta cheese.

Pimiento Cheese Meatballs

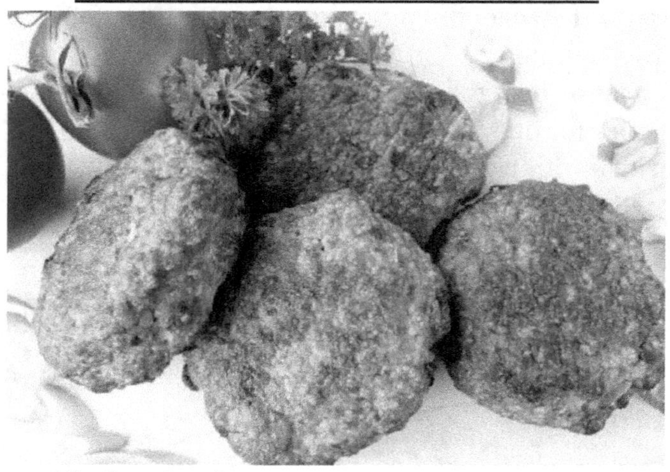

Yields Provided: 4 Servings
Nutritional Counts Per Serving:
- **Calories**: 660
- **Net Carbs**: 1 g
- **Total Fat Content**: 53 g
- **Protein**: 42 g

Ingredients Needed:
- Mayonnaise (.33 cup)
- Pimentos or pickled jalapeños (.25 cup)
- Paprika powder or chili powder (1 tsp.)
- Dijon mustard (1 tbsp.)
- Cayenne pepper (1 pinch)
- Grated cheddar cheese (4 oz.)

Ingredients Needed - The Meatballs:
- Ground beef (.25 oz.)
- Egg (1)
- Salt and pepper
- Butter - for frying (2 tbsp.)

How to Prepare:
1. Prepare all of the fixings for the cheese in a large mixing bowl and set aside for a few minutes.

2. Add the egg and the ground beef together and add to the rest of the ingredients. Sprinkle with the salt and pepper as desired.
3. Prepare the meatballs and fry them in oil or butter using the medium heat setting until they're done.
4. Serve with a salad of your choice.

Slow-Cooked Chuck Steak

Yields Provided: 8 Servings
Nutritional Counts Per Serving:
- **Calories:** 667
- **Net Carbs:** 3 g
- **Total Fat Content:** 33 g
- **Protein:** 79 g

Ingredients Needed:
- Chuck steak (4.5 lb.)
- Celery stalks (4)
- Carrots (3)
- Garlic cloves (2)
- Beef stock (2 cups)
- Red wine (1 cup)
- Pepper and salt (as desired)

How to Prepare:
1. Pour one inch of water into the cooker. Add the roast and prepare on the high setting for four hours. Slice the veggies and toss them around the roast.
2. Empty the wine and broth over the meat and add all of the spices.
3. Simmer for four more hours on the high setting.
4. Slice the steak into 8 servings and serve with the veggies.

Slow-Cooked London Broil

Yields Provided: 4 Servings
Nutritional Counts Per Serving:
- **Calories**: 409
- **Net Carbs**: 2.5 g
- **Total Fat Content**: 18 g
- **Protein**: 47 g

Ingredients Needed:
- Minced garlic (2 tsp.)
- London broil (2 lb.)
- Onion powder (2 tsp.)
- Dijon mustard (1 tbsp.)
- Reduced sugar ketchup (2 tbsp.)
- Coconut Aminos/soy sauce substitute (2 tbsp.)
- Coffee (.5 cup)
- Chicken broth (.5 cup)
- White wine (.25 cup)

How to Prepare:
1. Arrange the beef in the cooker. Cover both sides with the mustard, soy sauce, ketchup, and minced garlic.
2. Pour the liquid components into the cooker and give it a sprinkle of the onion powder.
3. Cook for four to six hours.
4. When the timer buzzes, shred the meat. Combine with the juices and serve.

Steak Pinwheels

Yields Provided: 6 Servings

Nutritional Counts Per Serving:

- **Calories**: 414
- **Net Carbs**: 2 g
- **Total Fat Content**: 20 g
- **Protein**: 55 g

Ingredients Needed:

- Flank steak (2 lb.)
- Mozzarella cheese (8 oz. pkg.)
- Spinach (1 bunch - 1.75 cups approx.)

How to Prepare:

1. Heat the oven to reach 350° Fahrenheit.
2. Slice the steak into six portions and remove all of the 'hard' fat. Beat until thin with a mallet.
3. Shred the cheese using a food processor and sprinkle the steak. Roll it up and tie with a piece of cooking twine or a skewer.
4. Line the pan with the pinwheels and place it on a layer of spinach. Bake until done (25 min.).

Jamaican Jerk Pork Roast

Yields Provided: 12 Servings
Nutritional Counts Per Serving:
- **Calories**: 282
- **Net Carbs**: 0 g
- **Total Fat Content**: 20 g
- **Protein**: 23 g

Ingredients Needed:
- Olive oil (1 tbsp.)
- Pork shoulder (4 lb.)
- Broth or beef stock (.5 cup)
- Jamaican Jerk spice blend (.25 cup)
- *Also Needed:* Dutch oven/regular oven

How to Prepare:
1. Rub the roast well using the oil, and coat with the jerk spice blend.
2. Use the Dutch oven to sear the roast on all sides. Add the beef broth.
3. Cover the pot and simmer for about four hours using the low heat setting. (You can also bake it for 3 hours at 375° Fahrenheit.)
4. Shred and serve.

Keto Pork Kabobs

Yields Provided: 4 Servings
Nutritional Counts Per Serving:
- **Net Carbs**: 3 g
- **Total Fat Content**: 9 g
- **Protein**: 34 g

Ingredients Needed:
- Water (1 tbsp.)
- Medium green pepper (1)
- Crushed red pepper (.5 tsp.)
- Squared pork for kebabs (1 lb.)
- Hot sauce (2 tsp.)
- Sunflower seed butter (3 tbsp.)
- Minced garlic (1 tbsp.)
- Keto-friendly soy sauce/Tamari sauce (1 tbsp.)

How to Prepare:
1. Heat the oven or grill using the broil or the high-heat setting.
2. In a processor or blender, combine the water with the red pepper, soy sauce, garlic, butter, and hot sauce.
3. Slice the pork into squares. Cover with the marinade and rest for 1 hour.
4. Chop the peppers to fit the skewer. Thread the skewers alternating the pork and peppers.
5. Broil using the high heat setting for five minutes per side.

Luau Pork with Cauli Rice

Yields Provided: 9 Servings
Nutritional Counts Per Serving:
- **Calories**: 182
- **Net Carbs**: 1 g
- **Total Fat Content**: 13 g
- **Protein**: 14 g

Ingredients Needed:
- Hickory smoked bacon (4 slices)
- Shoulder/pork roast (3 lb.)
- Hawaiian black lava sea salt (1-2 tbsp.)
- Minced garlic cloves (4-6)
- _Optional_: Hickory liquid smoke (2 tbsp.)

Ingredients Needed - The Rice:
- Homemade/organic chicken broth (2 tbsp.)
- Cauliflower (3 cups)
- Sea salt (0.125 tsp.)
- Garlic powder (.25 tsp.)

How to Prepare:
1. Set the slow cooker using the high setting. Layer the bacon slices and minced garlic in the bottom.
2. Pour the black lava salt in a small container. Poke holes in the roast and rub it with the salt and place it with the fatty side down. Add the liquid smoke and cover for two hours (high) or four to six hours (low). Bone-in may take eight to ten hours.
3. Remove the bones and shred the pork and continue cooking on low for 30 minutes to ensure the meat is done.
4. Begin making the rice at this point. You can microwave for five minutes or steam for 20 minutes on the stovetop. Add the slightly cooled product into the food processor along with the sea salt, garlic, and chicken broth. Process until it's a rice

texture. Serve on the side of the pork.

Pulled Pork Hash

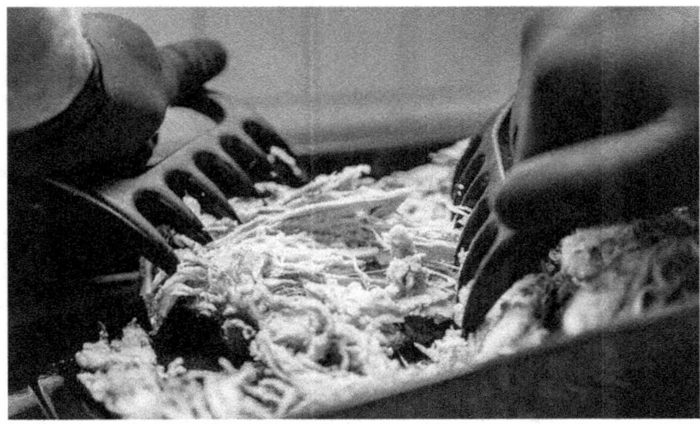

Yields Provided: 2 Servings
Nutritional Counts Per Serving:
- **Calories**: 354
- **Net Carbs**: 8 g
- **Total Fat Content**: 22 g
- **Protein**: 21 g

Ingredients Needed:
- Lard or fat of choice (2 tbsp.)
- Turnip (1)
- Black pepper (.25 tsp.)
- Salt (.25 tsp.)
- Paprika (.5 tsp.)
- Garlic powder (.25 tsp.)
- Brussels sprouts (3)
- Lacinato kale (about 2 leaves - 1 cup)
- Red onion (2 tbsp.)
- Pulled pork (3 oz.)
- Eggs (2)
- *Also Needed*: Large cast-iron skillet

How to Prepare:
1. Dice the turnip and slice the brussels sprouts into halves. Chop

the kale and dice the onion.

2. Warm up the oil in a skillet using the med-high temperature setting. Add the diced turnip and the spices.
3. Cook for approximately five minutes.
4. Stir in the rest of the vegetables and cook for another two to three minutes until they start to soften.
5. Add in the pork and cook for two more minutes.
6. Make two divots in the hash and crack in the eggs.
7. Cover and cook for three to five minutes just until the whites are set.

Stuffed Pork Chops

Yields Provided: 4 Servings
Nutritional Counts Per Serving:
- **Calories**: 778
- **Net Carbs**: 1 g
- **Total Fat Content**: 38 g
- **Protein**: 102 g

Ingredients Needed:
- Bacon (3 slices)
- Thick cut pork chops (4)
- Feta cheese (3 oz.)
- Blue cheese (3 oz.)
- Cream cheese (2 oz.)
- Green onion (.33 cup)
- Garlic powder (1 pinch)
- Black pepper & salt (as desired)

How to Prepare:
1. Program the oven temperature to 350° Fahrenheit.
2. Spritz a baking pan with a portion of cooking oil spray.
3. Prepare the bacon in a skillet - while reserving the grease and set aside.
4. Mix the feta and blue cheese. Blend in the onions and bacon. Next, add the cream cheese, and mix well.
5. Split the non-fat side of the pork, and add the cheese mixture, closing with a toothpick. Sprinkle using the garlic powder, salt, and pepper.
6. Sear with the bacon grease in the skillet for 1.5 minutes per side.
7. Arrange the chops on the baking pan.
8. Roast for 55 minutes.
9. Let the chops rest about three minutes.

Lamb Options

Lamb Chops with Herb Butter

Yields Provided: 4 Servings
Nutritional Counts Per Serving:
- **Calories**: 723
- **Net Carbs**: 0.3 g
- **Total Fat Content**: 62 g
- **Protein**: 43 g

Ingredients Needed:
- Unchilled lamb chops (8)
- Olive oil (1 tbsp.)
- Butter (1 tbsp.)
- Salt and pepper (as desired)

Ingredients Needed - For Serving:
- Herb butter (4 oz.)
- Lemon (1 in wedges)

How to Prepare:
1. Once the chops are at room temperature, slice the fat parts to eliminate it from curling up. Dust with the pepper and salt.
2. *For Grilling*: Lightly grease the fish with oil and place on the grill. *For Frying*: Use olive oil and butter in the pan.
3. Fry for 3 to 4 minutes. The center can be a little pink inside.
4. Serve with lemon wedges and herb butter (below).

Herb Butter

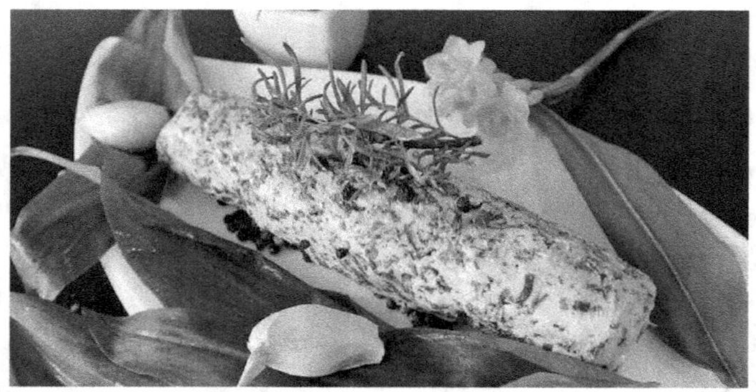

Yields Provided: 4 Servings
Nutritional Counts Per Serving:
- **Calories**: 258
- **Net Carbs**: 1 g
- **Total Fat Content**: 28 g
- **Protein**: 1 g

Ingredients Needed:
- Unchilled butter (5 oz.)
- Garlic clove (1 pressed)
- Garlic powder (.5 tbsp.)
- Finely chopped fresh parsley (4 tbsp.)
- Lemon juice (1 tsp.)
- Salt (.5 tsp.)

How to Prepare:
1. Finely chop the parsley and press the garlic clove. Mix all of the fixings in a small bowl.
2. Set aside for 15 minutes before serving.
3. If you prepare this ahead of time; you should store it in the refrigerator.

Lamb Curry

Yields Provided: 14 Servings
Nutritional Counts Per Serving:
- **Calories**: 480
- **Net Carbs**: 1 g
- **Total Fat Content**: 38 g
- **Protein**: 30 g

Ingredients Needed - Marinade:
- Ginger (2 tsp.)
- Garlic (3 cloves)
- Cumin ground (2 tsp.)
- Coriander ground (2 tsp.)
- Onion powder (1 tsp.)
- Cardamom ground (1 tsp.)
- Paprika ground (1 tsp.)
- Turmeric ground (1 tsp.)
- Kashmiri Chili Powder (1 tsp.)
- Olive oil (2 tbsp.)

Ingredients Needed - Curry
- Lamb shoulder diced (4 lb.)
- Ghee (3 tbsp.)
- Medium onion (1)
- Cinnamon (1 tsp.)
- Kashmiri Chili Powder (1 tsp.)
- Salt (2 tsp.)
- Pepper (1 tsp.)
- Heavy Cream (1 cup)
- Flaked almonds (.5 cup)
- Cilantro - roughly chopped (3 tbsp.)

How to Prepare:

1. Finely chop the ginger and garlic. Dice the onion.
2. Prepare the marinade. Thoroughly mix all marinade fixings.
3. Add the diced lamb and mix well. Marinate for one hour or overnight in the fridge.
4. Prepare the curry. Melt the ghee using medium heat. Toss in the onion, chili powder, and cinnamon. Sauté for three minutes.
5. Add the marinated lamb, pepper, and salt. Stir and simmer for 10 minutes before adding the cream. Reduce the heat setting to low. Simmer the curry, partially covered, for approximately one hour. At that time, check to see if it's done. If the lamb is tough, continue cooking until tender.
6. Take the pot from the pot. Simmer for another 10 minutes.
7. Add the flaked almonds and any extra seasoning.
8. Remove from the heat. Garnish with coriander and serve.

Roasted Leg of Lamb

Yields Provided: 2 Servings
Nutritional Counts Per Serving:
- **Calories:** 223
- **Net Carbs:** 1 g
- **Total Fat Content:** 14 g
- **Protein:** 22 g

Ingredients Needed:
Reduced-sodium beef broth (.5 cup)
Leg of lamb (2 lb.)
Chopped garlic cloves (6)
Fresh rosemary leaves (1 tbsp.)
Black pepper (1 tsp.)
Salt (2 tsp.)

How to Prepare:
Grease a baking pan and set the oven temperature at 400° Fahrenheit.
Arrange the lamb in the pan and add the broth and seasonings.
Roast 30 minutes and lower the heat setting to 350° Fahrenheit.
Continue cooking for about one hour or until done.
Let the lamb stand about 20 minutes before slicing to serve.

Other Options

Garlic Parmesan Sausage Skillet

Yields Provided: 6 Servings
Nutritional Counts Per Serving:
- **Calories:** 515
- **Net Carbs:** 8.4 g
- **Total Fat Content:** 45.7 g
- **Protein:** 16.6 g

Ingredients Needed:
- Olive oil (.25 cup)
- Brussels sprouts (8)
- Turnip (1)
- Large cremini mushrooms (4)
- Bell pepper (1)
- Zucchini (1)
- Yellow squash (1)
- Cherry tomatoes (.5 cup)
- Onion (.5 of 1)
- Roasted Garlic Kiolbassa (13 oz. pkg.)

Ingredients Needed - Parmesan Cream Sauce
- Butter (1 tbsp.)
- Roasted garlic (4 cloves)
- Cream cheese (2 oz.)
- Heavy cream (1 cup + 2 tbsp.)
- Grated parmesan cheese (.5 cup)

How to Prepare:

1. Slice the mushrooms and sprouts into halves. Mash the cloves and sprouts into halves. Dice the turnips and peppers.
2. Cut the zucchini and squash into half-moons. Cut the onion into quarters.
3. Warm the oil in a large cast-iron skillet using the med-high heat setting.
4. Once hot, add the sprouts with the cut-side down in the skillet. Also, add the turnips and simmer for 8-10 minutes until crispy.
5. Add the sausage and cook for 4-5 minutes until the kielbasa is starting to brown. Stir in the rest of the veggies, salt, and pepper. Cook for 10 minutes, stirring occasionally before removing and setting aside.
6. Mix in the butter with the heavy cream and roasted garlic. Simmer for 4 to 5 minutes until the cream is slightly reduced.
7. Stir in the cream cheese until just melted. Whisk in the parmesan cheese. Simmer until thickened. Add the mixtures together and serve.

Chapter 8: Side Dishes

Asparagus & Garlic

Yields Provided: 4 Servings
Nutritional Counts Per Serving:
- **Calories**: 61
- **Net Carbs**: 2 g
- **Total Fat Content**: 6 g
- **Protein**: 1 g

Ingredients Needed:
- Minced garlic (1 tbsp.)
- Fresh asparagus (1 bunch)
- Butter (2 tbsp.)

How to Prepare:
1. Rinse the asparagus and separate each of the stalks. Boil them for 2 to 3 minutes. Drain and chill in a dish of cold water.
2. Warm up the garlic and butter in a skillet. Fry the asparagus with them until browned and serve.

Broccoli & Cheese Casserole

Yields Provided: 5 Servings
Nutritional Counts Per Serving:
- **Calories**: 113
- **Net Carbs**: 2 g
- **Total Fat Content**: 9 g
- **Protein**: 6 g

Ingredients Needed:
- Broccoli florets (2 cups)
- Chopped onion (1 tbsp.)
- Fresh eggs (4)
- Mozzarella (.5 cup)
- Black pepper (.5 tsp.)
- Butter (2 tbsp.)

How to Prepare:
1. Warm the oven in advance to 350° Fahrenheit. Lightly grease a baking dish and set it aside for now.
2. Melt the margarine in a saucepan. Add the onion and sauté until translucent. Whisk the eggs and add to the onion. Dust using the pepper and salt.
3. Place the florets in the prepared container and add the egg fixings.
4. Sprinkle with cheese and bake for about 13 minutes or until set.
5. Set aside on a cooling rack to cool a few minutes before serving.

<u>Cauliflower Mac & Cheese</u>

Yields Provided: 4 Servings
Nutritional Counts Per Serving:
- **Calories:** 294
- **Net Carbs:** 7 g
- **Total Fat Content:** 23 g
- **Protein:** 11 g

Ingredients Needed:
- Butter (3 tbsp.)
- Cauliflower (1 head)
- Cheddar cheese (1 cup)
- Black pepper & sea salt (as desired)
- Unsweetened almond milk (.25 cup)
- Heavy cream (.25 cup)

How to Prepare:
1. Dice the cauliflower into small florets and shred the cheese.
2. Program the oven temperature setting to 450° Fahrenheit ahead of time.
3. Use a piece of aluminum foil or parchment paper to line a baking sheet.
4. Melt 2 tbsp. of butter. Toss in the florets and butter. Give it a shake of pepper and salt. Place the cauliflower on the baking pan and roast 10 to 15 minutes.
5. Warm the rest of the butter, milk, heavy cream, and cheese in a microwave or double boiler.
6. Pour in the cheese and serve.

Garlic Parmesan Fried Eggplant

Yields Provided: 6 Servings
Nutritional Counts Per Serving:
- **Calories**: 271
- **Net Carbs**: 6 g
- **Total Fat Content**: 22 g
- **Protein**: 12 g

Ingredients Needed:
- Large egg (1)
- Eggplant (1 medium)
- Garlic powder (2 tsp.)
- Salt divided (1 tsp.)
- Parmesan cheese (1 cup)
- Almond flour (1 cup)
- Coconut oil or butter (.5 cup)
- Pepper (.5 tsp.)

How to Prepare:
1. Slice the eggplant into .5-inch slices. Dust with .5 tsp. of the salt. Wait for about 30 minutes. Dab it dry using a paper towel and add to a baking sheet (single-layered).
2. Whisk the egg in one bowl.
3. In another container, whisk the salt, pepper, garlic powder, parmesan, and almond flour.
4. Heat 1-2 tablespoons of butter/oil using the medium heat temperature setting.
5. Dip the slices of eggplant in the egg, shake off the excess, and dredge in the almond flour concoction. Shake off the excess.
6. Fry the prepared slices in a skillet, browning until each side is browned and crispy. Drain on towels before serving.

Chapter 9: Appetizers

Air Fryer - Bacon-Wrapped Chicken

Yields Provided: 3 Servings
Nutritional Counts Per Serving:
- **Calories**: 364
- **Net Carbs**: 0.6 g
- **Total Fat Content**: 26 g
- **Protein**: 31 g

Ingredients Needed:
- Breast of chicken (1)
- Unsmoked bacon (6 strips)
- Soft garlic cheese (1 tbsp.)

How to Prepare:
1. Slice the chicken into six pieces. Spread the garlic cheese over each bacon strip. Add a piece of chicken to each one.
2. Roll and secure with a toothpick.
3. Let the Air Fryer warm up for three to four minutes.
4. Arrange the wraps in the hot fryer and cook 15 minutes for a quick snack at any time.

Bacon-Wrapped Mozzarella Sticks

Yields Provided: 2 Servings

Nutritional Counts Per Serving:
- **Calories**: 103
- **Net Carbs**: 1 g
- **Total Fat Content**: 9 g
- **Protein**: 7 g

Ingredients Needed:
- Thick bacon (2 slices)
- Frigo cheese head mozzarella cheese sticks (1)
- Coconut oil for frying
- Low-sugar pizza sauce for the dip
- Toothpicks

How to Prepare:
1. Warm the oil to 350° Fahrenheit in a deep fryer.
2. Slice the cheese stick in half. Wrap with bacon and secure it closed using a toothpick.
3. it
4. Drain on a layer of paper towels to cool. Serve with the sauce.

Cheese-Stuffed Bacon-Wrapped Hot Dogs

Yields Provided: 6 Servings
Nutritional Counts Per Serving:
- **Calories**: 283
- **Net Carbs**: 2.1 g
- **Total Fat Content**: 19.3 g
- **Protein**: 13.6 g

Ingredients Needed:
- Bacon (12 slices)
- Large beef hot dogs (6)
- Onion (.5 tsp.)
- Garlic (.5 tsp.)
- Pepper & salt (to your liking)
- Cheddar cheese (2 oz.)

How to Prepare:
1. Program the oven temperature to 400° Fahrenheit.
2. Slice each of the hot dogs (not all the way through) and insert the cheese.
3. Wrap the hot dogs/chicken with two bacon slices each and secure with a toothpick.
4. Add the seasoning to a dish and roll the dogs through it.
5. Bake 35 to 40 minutes.
6. Serve and enjoy with your favorite side dishes or as a snack.
7. *Note:* You can adjust the time and cook them as using small chunks for a variation.

Mortadella & Brie Plate

Yields Provided: 2 Servings
Nutritional Counts Per Serving:
- **Calories**: 1118
- **Net Carbs**: 6 g
- **Total Fat Content**: 103 g
- **Protein**: 40g

Ingredients Needed:
- Italian mortadella sausage (9 oz.)
- Brie cheese or Camembert cheese (5 oz.)
- Anchovies (.66 oz.)
- Green pesto (2 tbsp.)
- Black olives (10)
- Arugula lettuce (6 oz.)
- Keto-friendly mayo (.5 cup)
- Leaves of fresh basil (10)

How to Prepare:
1. Arrange the thinly sliced mortadella, anchovies, cheese, olives, pesto, and keto-friendly mayo on a platter.
2. Serve with the arugula and fresh basil.
3. _Note_: Mortadella is a large sausage or lunch meat made from pork.

Pita Pizza

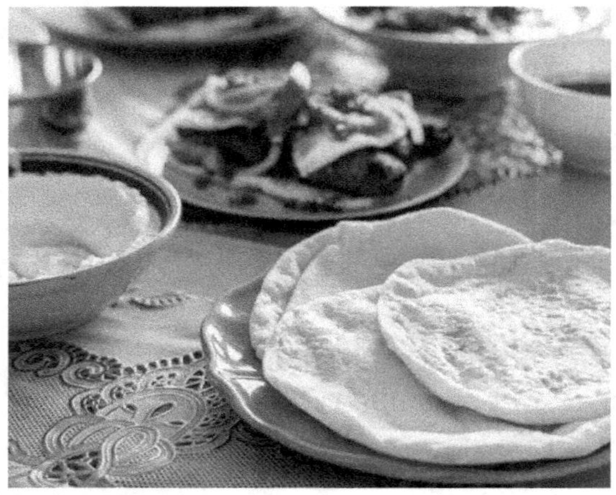

Yields Provided: 2 Servings
Nutritional Counts Per Serving:
- **Calories**: 250
- **Net Carbs**: 4 g
- **Total Fat Content**: 19 g
- **Protein**: 13 g

Ingredients Needed:
- Marinara sauce (.5 cup)
- Low-carb pita (1)
- Cheddar cheese (2 oz.)
- Pepperoni (14 slices)
- Roasted red peppers (1 oz.)

How to Prepare:
1. Set the oven temperature setting to 450° Fahrenheit.
2. Slice the pita in half and place onto a foil-lined baking tray. Rub with a bit of oil, and toast for one to two minutes.
3. Pour the sauce over the bread. Sprinkle using the cheese and other toppings. Bake for another five minutes or until the cheese melts.
4. Remove from the oven and let it cool thoroughly.

Salmon & Cream Cheese Bites

Yields Provided: 36 Servings
Nutritional Counts Per Serving:
- **Calories**: 32
- **Net Carbs**: 0.4 g
- **Total Fat Content**: 2.2 g
- **Protein**: 2 g

Ingredients Needed:
- Salt (.5 tsp.)
- Cream or milk (1 cup)
- Eggs (6 medium)
- Dried dill (.5 tsp.)
- Cream cheese (.33 cup)
- Shredded cheese (.5 cup)
- Fresh/smoked salmon slices (1.8 oz.)
- *Also Needed*: Mini muffin trays or silicone molds

How to Prepare:
1. Whisk the salt, eggs, and milk in a large measuring cup.
2. Fold in the smoked salmon, shredded cheese, and diced cream cheese.
3. Pour into the molds and bake for 10-15 minutes at 350° Fahrenheit.
4. Cool before removing to serve.

Sweet Choices

Choco Mug Brownie

Yields Provided: 1 Serving
Nutritional Counts Per Serving:
- **Calories:** 207
- **Net Carbs:** 9.5 g
- **Total Fat Content:** 16 g
- **Protein:** 12 g

Ingredients Needed:
- Chocolate protein powder (1 scoop)
- Cocoa powder (1 tbsp.)
- Baking powder (.5 tsp.)
- Almond milk (.25 cup)

How to Prepare:
1. Prepare a mug using the protein powder, cocoa, and baking powder.
2. Pour the milk into the mug and stir.
3. Microwave for about 30 seconds and serve.

Chocolate Biscotti

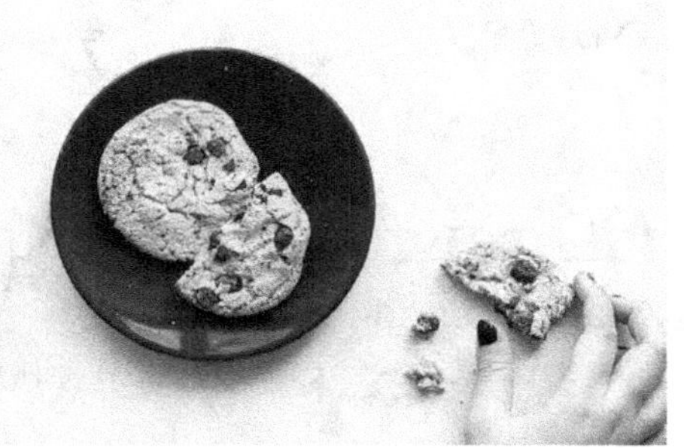

Yields Provided: 15 Servings
Nutritional Counts Per Serving:
- **Calories**: 82
- **Net Carbs**: 2 g
- **Total Fat Content**: 7 g
- **Protein**: 3 g

Ingredients Needed:
- Large egg (1)
- Monk fruit sweetener or erythritol (.25 cup)
- Stevia concentrated powder (.25 tsp.)
- Softened butter (.25 cup)
- Vanilla extract (.5 tsp.)
- Almond flour (1.75 cups)
- Xanthan gum (.25 tsp.)
- Unsweetened cocoa (.5 cup)
- Baking soda (.5 tsp.)
- Sea salt (.25 tsp.)
- Cinnamon (1 tsp.)
- *Optional:* Sugar-free chocolate chips
- *Optional:* Chopped nuts

How to Prepare:
1. Set the oven to reach 325° Fahrenheit.

2. Mix the butter with the egg, stevia, granular sweetener, and vanilla.

3. In another container, sift or whisk all the dry fixings and mix until well incorporated.

4. Combine the wet and dry fixings, stirring as you go. Chocolate chips or nuts can be mixed in at this time.

5. Prepare the ball of dough. Arrange the dough ball on a layer of parchment baking paper, silicone baking mat or cookie sheet. Shape the dough into a long flat log.

6. Bake for approximately 18 to 20 minutes. Transfer from the oven and lower the heat setting to 275° Fahrenheit. Cool for about 10 minutes. Slice into thin strips about .5-inch wide.

7. Arrange the slices on the cookie sheet. Bake until crispy for about 20 minutes to half an hour.

Chocolate Zucchini Cookies

Yields Provided: 12 Servings
Nutritional Counts Per Serving:
- **Calories**: 140
- **Net Carbs**: 2 g
- **Total Fat Content**: 13 g
- **Protein**: 3 g

Ingredients Needed:
- Zucchini (1 cup)
- Salt (.5 tsp.)
- Cinnamon (.25 tsp.)
- Almond flour (1 cup)
- Baking soda (.5 tsp.)
- Coconut flour (.25 cup)
- Cacao powder or unsweetened cocoa powder (.25 cup)
- Monk fruit sweetener or raw honey (.5 cup)
- Butter flavored coconut oil or ghee (.33 cup)
- Vanilla extract (1 tsp.)
- Large egg yolk (1)
- *Optional*: Sugar-free chocolate chips or dark chocolate pieces (.25 cup)

How to Prepare:
1. Grate the zucchini, and wrap it in a towel to squeeze out excess liquid.
2. Whisk the dry fixings (salt, almond flour, cacao powder, coconut flour, cinnamon, and baking soda). Put it to the side for now.
3. In a glass mixing bowl, melt the coconut oil/ghee. Whisk in the sweetener, egg yolk, and vanilla extract.
4. Stir the zucchini into the sweetened mixture and combine it with the dry ingredients. Fold in chocolate if using.
5. Shape the dough into tbsp.-sized balls by rolling in your hands.
6. Flatten each ball out and top each with a piece or two of chocolate.

7. Bake at 350° Fahrenheit for 10 to 12 minutes. Serve.

Cinnamon Coconut Chips

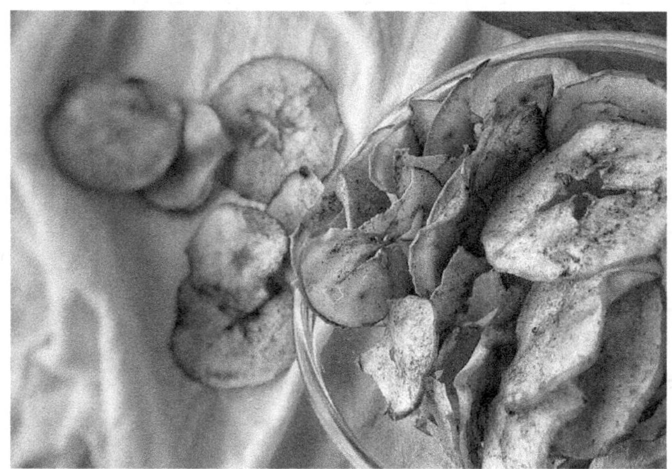

Yields Provided: 2 Servings

Nutritional Counts Per Serving:

- **Calories**: 228
- **Net Carbs**: 8 g
- **Total Fat Content**: 21 g
- **Protein**: 2 g

Ingredients Needed:

- Cinnamon (.25 tsp.)
- Sea salt (.25 tsp.)
- Unsweetened coconut chips (1 cup)

How to Prepare:

1. Whisk the salt and cinnamon together.
2. Use the medium heat temperature setting to warm a skillet (2 min.).
3. Stir in the chips, stirring until lightly browned.
4. Toss using the salt and cinnamon mixture before serving.

Orange Cream Cheese Cookies & Nuts

Yields Provided: 18 Servings
Nutritional Counts Per Serving:
- **Calories:** 200
- **Net Carbs:** 2 g
- **Total Fat Content:** 19 g
- **Protein:** 3 g

Ingredients Needed:
- Softened butter (.75 cup)
- Eggs (3)
- Coconut flour (.5 cup)
- Baking powder (1.5 tsp.)
- Monk fruit sweetener (.75 cup)
- Baking soda (.25 tsp.)
- Sugar-free dried cranberries (.25 cup)
- Macadamia nuts chopped (.5 cup)
- Dried grated orange zest (1.5 tsp.)

How to Prepare:
1. In a mixing container, beat the sweetener with the eggs and butter until well combined.
2. Whisk or sift the coconut flour, baking powder, and soda. Beat on the low setting or with a spoon until fully mixed.
3. Fold in the berries, orange zest, and nuts.
4. Shape into rounds and arrange on the cookie sheet.
5. Arrange the cookies a minimum of one inch apart for baking on a parchment-lined cookie sheet. Press each mound down slightly to flatten.
6. Bake at 350° Fahrenheit until edges have started to brown or for eight to ten minutes. Cool on a cooling rack.
7. Enjoy right out of the fridge for a week or they can be frozen for longer storage.

Peanut Butter & Coconut Balls

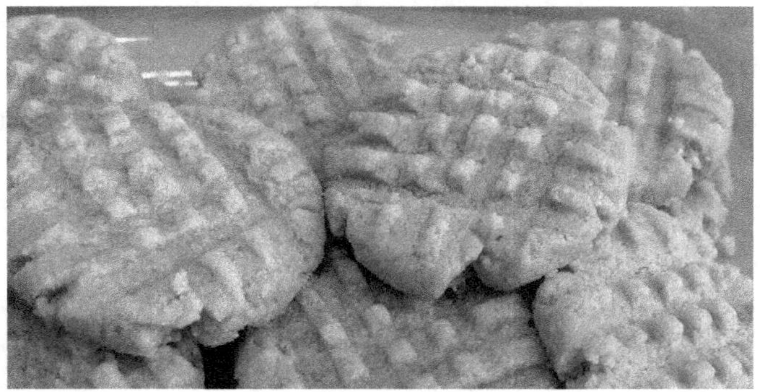

Yields Provided: 15 Servings
Nutritional Counts Per Serving:
- **Calories**: 35
- **Net Carbs**: 0.9 g
- **Total Fat Content**: 3.2 g
- **Protein**: 0.98 g

Ingredients Needed:
- Powdered erythritol (2.5 tsp.)
- Creamy peanut butter – keto-friendly (3 tbsp.)
- Unsweetened cocoa powder (3 tsp.)
- Almond flour (2 tsp.)
- Unsweetened coconut flakes (.5 cup)

How to Prepare:
1. Combine the peanut butter, cocoa, erythritol, and flour. Place in the freezer for one hour.
2. Spoon out a small spoon-size of the peanut butter mix. Roll into the flakes until it is covered.
3. Refrigerate overnight for the best results.

Pistachio Cookies

Yields Provided: 16 Servings
Nutritional Counts Per Serving:
- **Calories**: 135
- **Net Carbs**: 2 g
- **Total Fat Content**: 12 g
- **Protein**: 4 g

Ingredients Needed:
- Melted butter (6 tbsp.)
- Chopped pistachios (.5 cup)
- Erythritol (.5 cup)
- Almond flour (2 cups)

How to Prepare:
1. Whisk all of the fixings in a mixing container.
2. Shape the dough into a long roll. Cover with a sheet of plastic wrap.
3. Place in the fridge for about 30 minutes. Unwrap and slice into 16 portions.
4. Bake for 12 to 15 minutes. Cool slightly and serve.

Salty Choices

Bacon Cheddar Cheese Crisps

Yields Provided: 3 Servings
Nutritional Counts Per Serving:
- **Calories**: 150
- **Net Carbs**: 1.1 g
- **Total Fat Content**: 11.8 g
- **Protein**: 0.7 g

Ingredients Needed:
- Cooked bacon (3 strips)
- Shredded cheddar cheese (1 cup)

How to Prepare:
1. Set the oven ahead of time to 350° Fahrenheit.
2. Prepare a baking tin with a sheet of parchment paper.
3. Pour about one tablespoon of the cheese onto the tray for each serving. Break the bacon to bits and add to the piles of cheese.
4. Bake for 5 to 8 minutes and let cool. Blot the grease away with a paper towel before serving.

Bacon Knots

Yields Provided: 12 Servings

Nutritional Counts Per Serving:

- **Calories:** 442
- **Net Carbs:** 1.3 g
- **Total Fat Content:** 33 g
- **Protein:** 30 g

Ingredients Needed:

- Raw bacon (16 slices)
- Shredded parmesan (.25 cup)
- Minced garlic (4 cloves)
- Minced parsley (1 tbsp.)
- Pepper & Salt (as desired)

How to Prepare:

1. Straighten one slice of bacon. Tie it into a knot.
2. Take another slice, and tie another knot around the first one. Continue until done.
3. Place the chain on a parchment-lined baking tin.
4. Warm up the oven to reach 400° Fahrenheit.
5. Sprinkle the bacon with garlic. Bake for 15 minutes.
6. When crispy, sprinkle with the parsley and cheese.
7. Bake for one more minute. Break apart and serve.

<u>Bacon-Wrapped Mushrooms</u>

Yields Provided: 12 Servings
Nutritional Counts Per Serving:

- **Calories:** 275
- **Net Carbs:** 1.6 g
- **Total Fat Content:** 26.4 g
- **Protein:** 8 g

Ingredients Needed:

- Strips of bacon (25)
- Portobello or white mushrooms (25)
- Black pepper & salt (to your liking)
- *Also Needed*: Toothpicks

How to Prepare:

1. Warm up the oven to reach 400° Fahrenheit.
2. Remove the stems from the mushrooms and wrap each cap with a bacon strip. Securely close with the toothpick.
3. Arrange each of the prepared treats on the prepared pan.
4. Bake for 15 minutes. Place on paper towels to drain. Serve or store for later.

Beef Pizza

Yields Provided: 4 Servings
Nutritional Counts Per Serving:
- **Calories**: 610
- **Net Carbs**: 2 g
- **Total Fat Content**: 45 g
- **Protein**: 44 g

Ingredients Needed:
- Large eggs (2)
- Ground beef (20 oz.)
- Pepperoni (28 slices)
- Shredded cheddar cheese (.5 cup)
- Pizza sauce (.5 cup)
- Mozzarella cheese (4 oz.)
- *Also Needed*: 1 Cast iron skillet

How to Prepare:
1. Combine the eggs, beef, and seasonings. Toss into a skillet to form the crust. Bake until done (15 min.).
2. Take it out of the oven and add the sauce, cheese, and toppings.
3. Place the pizza in the oven at 400° Fahrenheit for three or four minutes until the cheese has melted. Remove and serve.

Cheese Chips

Yields Provided: 4 Servings
Nutritional Counts Per Serving:
- **Calories**: 191
- **Net Carbs**: 0.1 g
- **Total Fat Content**: 16 g
- **Protein**: 16 g

Ingredients Needed:
- Cheddar or Edam cheese slices (8 oz.)
- Hot paprika (.5 tsp.)

How to Prepare:
1. Set the oven temperature setting at 400° Fahrenheit.
2. Place the cheese slices on a parchment paper-lined baking tin.
3. Sprinkle using the paprika.
4. Bake for 8 to 10 minutes. Cool to serve.

Cheese Puffs

Yields Provided: 3 Servings
Nutritional Counts Per Serving:
- **Calories:** 167
- **Net Carbs:** 0.2 g
- **Total Fat Content:** 14 g
- **Protein:** 10 g

Ingredients Needed:
- Brie Cheese (5.33 oz.)

How to Prepare:
1. Slice the cheese into cubes about .5 inches thick. Remove the white edge.
2. Arrange a few slices on a parchment paper-lined platter.
3. Place in the microwave for one to two minutes using the full-power setting.
4. Watch carefully, making only a few at a time.
5. Cool before serving and spice to your liking.

Cheese Wraps

Yields Provided: 4 Servings
Nutritional Counts Per Serving:
- **Calories**: 335
- **Net Carbs**: 2 g
- **Total Fat Content**: 31 g
- **Protein**: 13 g

Ingredients Needed:
- Butter (2 oz.)
- Cheddar/Edam/Provolone cheese slices (8 oz.)

How to Prepare:
1. Arrange the slices on a cutting board.
2. Thinly slice the butter and place in each of the slices.
3. Roll them up and sprinkle with your favorite spices for a quick snack.

Fried Queso Fresco

Yields Provided: 5 Servings
Nutritional Counts Per Serving:
- **Calories**: 307
- **Net Carbs**: 2.7 g
- **Total Fat Content**: 26 g
- **Protein**: 16 g

Ingredients Needed:
- Coconut oil (1 tbsp.)
- Queso fresco (1 lb.)
- Olive oil (.5 tbsp.)

How to Prepare:
1. Chop the cheese into cubes.
2. Heat each of the oils to the smoking point, and toss in the cheese.
3. Fry the cheese, flipping until well browned.
4. Remove and let the cheese rest to cool.
5. Drain on towels to remove the oil.

<u>Nut-Free Keto Crackers</u>

Yields Provided: 6 Servings - 4 crackers each
Nutritional Counts Per Serving:
- **Calories**: 407
- **Net Carbs**: 5 g
- **Total Fat Content**: 36 g
- **Protein**: 14 g

Ingredients Needed:
- Sunflower seeds - divided (.5 cup)
- Pumpkin seeds - divided (.5 cup)
- Sesame seeds (.33 cup)
- Ground flax seeds (2 tbsp.)
- Onion powder (.25 tsp.)
- Garlic powder (.25 tsp.)
- Salt (.5 tsp.)
- Egg (1)
- Butter or coconut oil - melted and cooled (2 tbsp.)

Ingredients Needed - Seasonings:
- Dried herbs; like rosemary - thyme and/or oregano
- Grated parmesan cheese + additional egg if parmesan is added (.33 - .5 cup)
- Oil-soaked sun-dried tomatoes (6)

How to Prepare:
1. Set the oven at 400° Fahrenheit.
2. Drain and roughly chop the tomatoes. Toss the sunflower seeds and pumpkin seeds into a food processor. Pulse until ground. Transfer the ground seeds to a large mixing bowl. Add the rest of the fixings. Add the seasonings at this time.
3. In a separate mixing container, using a fork, mix the egg and melted butter. Transfer the wet fixings to the bowl of dry fixings. Knead together until well-combined and a dough has

formed.

4. Roll the dough into a ball and place on a parchment-paper-lined plate. Transfer to the fridge to chill for 10 to 15 minutes.

5. Remove the dough from the refrigerator. Lay one piece of parchment paper down, placing the chilled dough in the center of the paper. Lay another piece of parchment paper down atop the dough. Lightly press down. Using a rolling pin, roll the dough until it is an even thin layer. Discard the top piece of parchment paper. Carefully slide a baking sheet beneath the parchment paper with the dough on top.

6. Form the dough into a rectangle, gently pushing the edges of dough against a knife to create straight edges.

7. Using a pizza cutter, score the dough (don't cut all the way through) to form 24 crackers.

8. Bake the crackers until golden brown, about 15 to 20 minutes. After baking, remove from oven and cut the crackers all the way through.

9. Cool the crackers to cool on the baking sheet for at least 30 minutes to harden and crisp up.

Olive Cheese Balls

Yields Provided: 12 Servings
Nutritional Counts Per Serving:
- **Calories:** 110
- **Net Carbs:** 5 g
- **Total Fat Content:** 8 g
- **Protein:** 4 g

Ingredients Needed:
- Pimento stuffed olives (24)
- Shredded cheddar cheese (1 cup)
- Softened butter (2 tbsp.)
- Keto-friendly flour of choice - ex. coconut or almond (.5 cup)
- Cayenne pepper (to your liking)

How to Prepare:
1. Warm up the oven to reach 400° Fahrenheit.
2. Combine the butter and cheese in a mixing container. Fold in the flour and mix combining with the pepper.
3. Wrap the mixture around each of the olives. Place on the cookie sheet.
4. Bake for about 15 minutes and serve or enjoy later.

Roasted Almonds

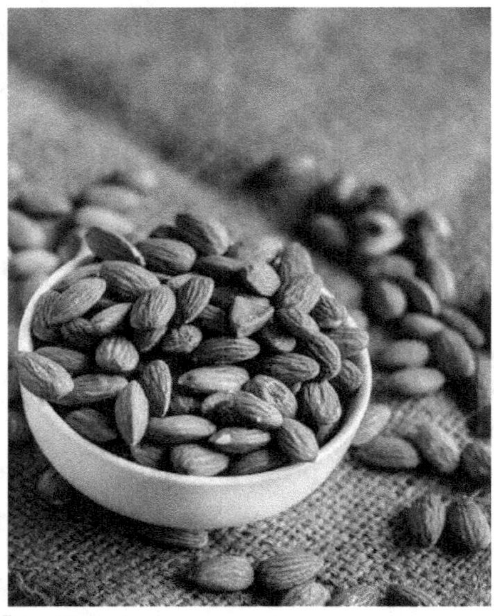

Yields Provided: 4 Servings
Nutritional Counts Per Serving:
- **Calories:** 342
- **Net Carbs:** 11.5 g
- **Total Fat Content:** 31 g
- **Protein:** 10 g

Ingredients Needed:
- Blanched almonds (2 cups)
- Paprika (1 tsp.)
- Rosemary (2 tbsp.)
- Salt (1 tsp.)
- Olive oil (2 tbsp.)

How to Prepare:
1. Toast the almonds in a pan using the med-high temperature setting.
2. Lower to medium-low and stir in paprika, rosemary, and salt.
3. Continue cooking for about three minutes before serving.

Roasted Pumpkin Seeds

Yields Provided: 8 Servings
Nutritional Counts Per Serving:
- **Calories**: 305
- **Net Carbs**: 6 g
- **Total Fat Content**: 25 g
- **Protein**: 12 g

Ingredients Needed:
- Cumin (.25 tsp.)
- Paprika (.5 tsp.)
- Raw pumpkin seeds (2 cups)
- Garlic salt (1 tsp.)
- Ghee (1 tsp.)
- Coconut aminos (1 tsp.)

How to Prepare:
1. Set the oven to reach 300º Fahrenheit.
2. Combine the cumin, paprika, garlic salt, coconut aminos, and ghee, with the pumpkin seeds.
3. In a single layer, add the seeds and toss with the ghee/oil.
4. Bake until crispy or for about one hour.

Slow-Roasted Cashews

Yields Provided: 4 Servings
Nutritional Counts Per Serving:
- **Calories**: 205
- **Net Carbs**: 14 g
- **Total Fat Content**: 16 g
- **Protein**: 5 g

Ingredients Needed:
- Cashews (1 cup)
- Cinnamon (2 tbsp.)
- Water (1 cup)

How to Prepare:
1. Pour the cashews and water into a container to soak overnight.
2. Drain and dry on a layer of paper towels.
3. Heat the oven to reach 200° Fahrenheit.
4. Toss the cashews on a baking tray and sprinkle using the cinnamon.
5. Roast for three hours. Cool before serving.

Chapter 11: Desserts

Banana Split Cheesecake

Yields Provided: 20 Servings

Nutritional Counts Per Serving:
- **Calories**: 302
- **Net Carbs**: 7 g
- **Total Fat Content**: 30 g
- **Protein**: 4 g

Ingredients Needed - For the Crust:
- Cinnamon (2 tsp.)
- Almond flour (3 cups)
- Swerve (.33 cup)
- Melted butter (1 cup)
- *Also Needed*: 9 x 13-inch pan

Ingredients Needed - For the Filling:
- Swerve confectioner's sugar (1 cup)
- Melted butter (1 cup)
- Cream cheese (16 oz.)

Ingredients Needed - For the Topping:
- Chopped banana (1)
- Sliced strawberries (2 pints)
- Lemon juice (1 tbsp.)
- Heavy whipping cream (2 cups)
- Gelatin (1.5 tsp.)
- Vanilla extract (1 tsp.)
- Swerve (3 tbsp.)
- Water (3 tbsp.)
- *Optional:* Chocolate sauce & Nuts

How to Prepare:
1. Combine the crust fixings, and press together in the pan.
2. Melt the butter and mix with the sweetener and cream cheese until creamy. Spread on top of the crust.
3. Combine the strawberries and banana in a mixing dish along with the lemon juice. Make the next layer.
4. Prepare the topping. Combine the whipping cream and gelatin in the water and beat well. Blend in the vanilla extract and sweetener. Whip until it is creamy to cover and make the next layer.
5. Top with the chocolate sauce and nuts if you like it that way.

**Blueberry Bar**

Yields Provided: 12 Servings
Nutritional Counts Per Serving:
- **Calories**: 385
- **Net Carbs**: 7 g
- **Total Fat Content**: 36 g
- **Protein**: 11 g

Ingredients Needed - For the Pecan Crust:
- Toasted pecans (1 cup)
- Almond flour (1 cup)
- Sukrin Gold powdered / Erythritol / Swerve (.33 cup)
- Whey protein isolate - Isopure (.25 cup)
- Melted butter (4 tbsp. - 2 oz.)
- *Also Needed*: 8x8 or 9x9-inch square baking pan

Ingredients Needed - For the Cake:
- Softened cream cheese (2 pkg. -16 oz.)
- Heavy whipping cream (.5 cup)
- Sukrin Icing Sugar or your choice (.66 cup/3 oz.)
- Vanilla extract (1 tbsp.)
- Stevia glycerite (.5 tsp.)

Ingredients Needed - For the Topping:
- Blueberries: Frozen or fresh (2 cups/10 oz.)
- Water (3 tbsp.)
- Lemon juice (1 tbsp.)
- Erythritol (3 tbsp. or more to taste)
- Nutmeg (1 pinch)

How to Prepare:
1. Toast the pecans and cool. Toss into a food processor to finely grind.
2. Gather the fixings. Butter or spray the bottom of a baking pan. Melt the 4 tablespoons of butter.
3. Prepare the Crust: Mix all of the dry fixings. Mix in melted

butter until it holds together when squeezed gently in your fist.

4. Scoop the crust mixture onto the baking pan and secure it with a layer of waxed paper over the crus. Press it firmly into the pan.

5. Prepare the Cheesecake Layer: Use a hand mixer to mix the cream cheese until smooth. Mix in the sweeteners and vanilla.

6. In another container, whisk the whipped cream until stiff.

7. Prepare in three batches. Start by folding the whipped cream into the sweetened cream cheese mixture. Spread the cheesecake fixings into the crust and chill in the fridge overnight.

8. Prepare the Topping: Put all of the fixings into a medium pan using the medium heat setting. Place a lid on the pot. Bring the mixture to a boil and lower to med-low or low. Simmer for about ten to fifteen minutes with the lid off until some of the blueberries burst and the sauce has thickened. Cool.

9. Pour the cooled sauce over the whole pan and cut into 12 portions or cut and spoon two to three tablespoons of the sauce over each bar.

Caramel Cake

Yields Provided: 12 Servings

Nutritional Counts Per Serving:
- **Calories**: 388
- **Net Carbs**: 4 g
- **Total Fat Content**: 35 g
- **Protein**: 10 g

Ingredients Needed:
- Almond flour (2.5 cups)
- Coconut flour (.25 cup)
- Unflavored whey protein powder (.25 cup)
- Salt (.5 tsp.)
- Baking powder (1 tbsp.)
- Softened butter (.5 cup)
- Swerve sweetener (.66 cup)
- Eggs - room temperature (4 large)
- Vanilla extract (1 tsp.)
- Almond milk (.75 cup)
- Sugar-free caramel sauce (2 batches)

How to Prepare - The Cake:
1. Set the oven to reach 325° Fahrenheit. Grease two 8-inch round cake pans. Cut a sheet of parchment to line the bottoms of the pans and grease the parchment as well.
2. Sift the coconut and almond flour, whey protein, salt, and baking powder.
3. Beat the butter and sweetener until light and fluffy. Beat in the eggs - one at a time and scrape down the beaters and bowl as needed. Stir in the vanilla extract.
4. Fold in the dry fixings in two additions; alternating with the almond milk. Beat until well combined.
5. Scoop the batter into the two cake pans; spreading it evenly to the edges. Smooth the tops and bake until the tops are firm to the touch (25 min.).
6. Place on the countertop to cool while in the pans. Then, flip

out onto a wire rack. Be sure to peel off the parchment paper if it sticks to the cake layers.

How to Prepare - Caramel Glaze:

1. Prepare a double batch of the Sugar-Free Caramel Sauce but *DO NOT* add the additional water at the end of the recipe. Be sure to use a large saucepan (at least 3-quarts) as it will bubble up.
2. Let the sauce cool down to room temperature. It should be quite thick at this point, but still pourable, and it will continue to thicken as it cools.
3. Place one layer of cake on a serving platter and pour about one-third of the caramel sauce on top. Carefully spread to the edges with an offset spatula and let sit another 10 to 15 minutes to thicken further.
4. Secure layer two and pour some of the caramel over the top, letting it drip down the sides, spreading it over the top and sides as you go. Continue until the top and sides are well covered. Alternatively, you can simply let it drip down the sides and not spread it over.
5. ***If your caramel is too thin and is dripping too much off the sides of the cake, you can whisk in a tablespoon or two of powdered Swerve to help thicken it up. If it gets too thick, you can gently rewarm it over low heat to thin it up again.

Cheesecake Pudding

Yields Provided: 4 Servings
Nutritional Counts Per Serving:
- **Calories**: 356
- **Net Carbs**: 5 g
- **Total Fat Content**: 36 g
- **Protein**: 5 g

Ingredients Needed:
- Cream cheese or Neufchatel cheese (1 block)
- Sour cream (.5 cup)
- Heavy whipping cream (.5 cup)
- Lemon juice (1 tsp.)
- Liquid stevia (20 drops)
- Vanilla extract (1 tsp.)

How to Prepare:
1. Microwave the cream cheese for 30 seconds or leave on the counter to soften for a few minutes before using it.
2. Whip the sour cream and whipping cream together with a mixer until soft peaks form. Combine with the rest of the fixings and whip until fluffy.
3. Portion into four dishes to chill. Place a layer of the wrap over the dish and store in the fridge.
4. When ready to eat, garnish with some berries if you like. If you add berries, be sure to add the carbs.

Chocolate Hazelnut Tarts

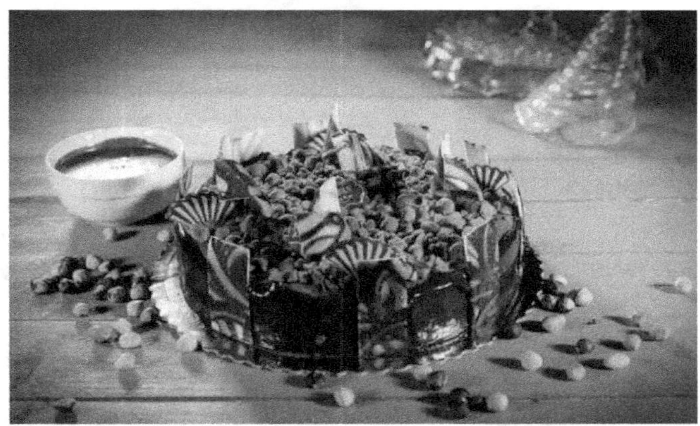

Yields Provided: 8 Servings
Nutritional Counts Per Serving:
- **Calories**: 223
- **Net Carbs**: 3 g
- **Total Fat Content**: 18 g
- **Protein**: 6 g

Ingredients Needed:
- Keto-friendly mini pie crusts (4)
- Melted coconut cream (2 tbsp.)
- Erythritol (as desired)
- Melted coconut oil (2 tbsp.)
- 100% chocolate - melted (2 oz.)
- Hazelnut butter (.25 cup)

How to Prepare:
1. Mix the coconut oil, coconut cream, chocolate, and erythritol together.
2. Pour 1 tbsp. of the hazelnut butter in each tart crust.
3. Next, pour the chocolate mixture on top while filling up the tart crust.
4. Refrigerate for two hours until solid.

Chocolate Lava Cake

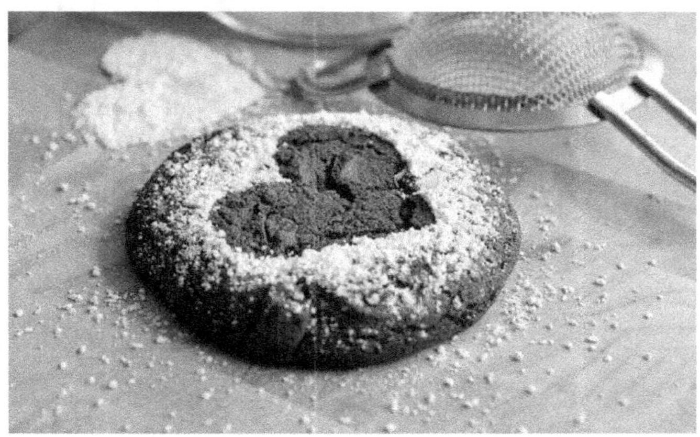

Yields Provided: 4 Servings
Nutritional Counts Per Serving:
- **Calories**: 189
- **Net Carbs**: 3 g
- **Total Fat Content**: 17 g
- **Protein**: 8 g

Ingredients Needed:
- Sugar-free chocolate sauce (.25 cup)
- Melted butter (.25 cup)
- Unsweetened cocoa powder (.5 cup)
- Eggs (4)
- Sea salt (.5 tsp.)
- Ground cinnamon (.5 tsp.)
- Pure vanilla extract (1 tsp.)
- Stevia (.25 cup)
- *Also Needed:* Ice cube tray & 4 ramekins

How to Prepare:
1. Pour 1 tablespoon of the chocolate sauce into 4 of the tray slots and freeze.

2. Warm up the oven to 350° Fahrenheit. Lightly grease the ramekins with butter or a spritz of oil.
3. Mix the salt, cinnamon, cocoa powder, and stevia until combined. Whisk in eggs – one at a time. Stir in the melted vanilla extract and butter.
4. Fill each of the ramekins halfway and add one of the frozen chocolates. Cover the rest of the container with the cake batter.
5. Bake for 13-14 minutes. When they're set, place on a wire rack to cool for about five minutes. Remove and put on a serving dish.
6. Enjoy by slicing its molten center.

Coconut Cream Brownies

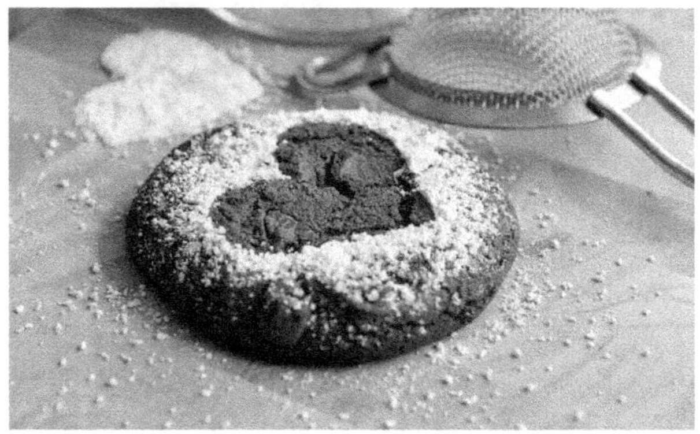

Yields Provided: 6 Servings
Nutritional Counts Per Serving:
- **Calories**: 175
- **Net Carbs**: 2 g
- **Total Fat Content**: 17 g
- **Protein**: 3 g

Ingredients Needed:
- Coconut cream (.33 cup)
- Melted coconut butter (.75 cup)
- Raw - unsweetened cocoa powder (.33 cup)
- Coconut flour (.33 cup)
- Melted butter or coconut oil (2 tbsp.)
- Stevia sugar substitute (.5 cup)
- Pure vanilla extract (1 tsp.)
- Sea salt (1 pinch)
- Egg (1)
- Baking soda (.25 tsp.)
- *Also Needed*: 3x9-inch loaf pan

How to Prepare:
1. Set the oven to reach 350° Fahrenheit.
2. Combine the flour, cocoa powder, stevia, salt, and baking

powder.

3. Whisk the coconut cream and butter in another container. Once combined, mix in the vanilla and whisked egg.
4. Combine all of the fixings well and add to the baking pan. Bake for 20 minutes. Once it's done, cool and slice into six equal squares.

Cranberry Bliss Cookies

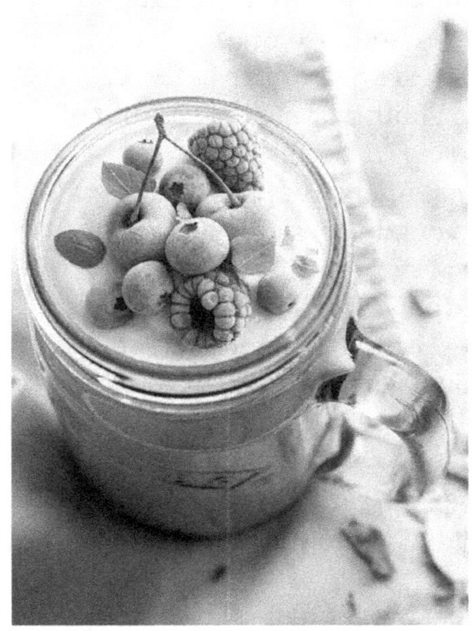

Yields Provided: 18 Servings
Nutritional Counts Per Serving:
- **Calories**: 145
- **Net Carbs**: 2 g
- **Total Fat Content**: 13 g
- **Protein**: 3 g

Ingredients Needed - For the Cookies:
- Almond flour (2 cups)
- Swerve Sweetener (.5 cup)
- Baking powder (1 tsp.)
- Ground ginger (.75 tsp.)
- Salt (.25 tsp.)
- Softened butter (6 tbsp.)
- Unchilled egg room (1 large)
- Vanilla extract (.5 tsp.)

- Fresh cranberries (.25 cup - chopped)

Ingredients Needed - For the Frosting:
- Cream cheese - softened (4 oz.)
- Powdered Swerve Sweetener (2 tbsp.)
- Melted cocoa butter or melted coconut oil (.5 oz.)
- Vanilla extract (.25 tsp.)
- Unsweetened finely chopped fresh cranberries (.25 cup) or freeze-dried cranberries crushed

Ingredients Needed - For the Drizzle:
- Cocoa butter melted/coconut oil (.5 oz.)
- Powdered Swerve sweetener (2 tbsp.)

How to Prepare:
1. Heat the oven to reach 325° Fahrenheit.
2. Prepare a large baking tray with a layer of parchment baking paper.
3. Whisk the baking powder, almond flour, salt, and ginger. In a large mixing container, mix the sweetener and butter until well combined. Fold in the vanilla extract and whisked egg.
4. Mix in the dry fixings and fold in the chopped cranberries.
5. Scoop and roll into one-inch balls. Press flat (.33-inch thickness) on the tin a few inches apart.
6. Bake 12 to 15 minutes until not quite firm to the touch. They will firm up as they sit. Cool in the pan.
7. *Prepare the Frosting:* Beat the cream cheese with the powdered sweetener until well combined. Melt and slowly add the cocoa butter and vanilla extract.
8. Frost the cookies. Decorate with a sprinkle of dried cranberries.
9. Whisk the powdered sweetener and melted cocoa butter until smooth. Drizzle over the cookies and let them sit for half an hour before serving.

Raspberry Coconut Cake – Slow-Cooked

Yields Provided: 10 Servings
Nutritional Counts Per Serving:
- **Calories**: 362
- **Net Carbs**: 7 g
- **Total Fat Content**: 32 g
- **Protein**: 10 g

Ingredients Needed:
- Unsweetened shredded coconut (1 cup)
- Almond flour (2 cups)
- Swerve sweetener (.75- 1 cup)
- Large eggs (4)
- Powdered egg whites (.25 cup)
- Salt (.25 tsp.)
- Baking soda (2 tsp.)
- Melted coconut oil (.5 cup)
- Raspberries – fresh or frozen (1 cup)
- Coconut extract (1 tsp.)
- Almond or coconut milk (.75 cup)
- Sugar-free dark chocolate chips (.33 cup)
- Coconut oil or favorite cooking spray
- _Suggested_: 6-quart size

How to Prepare:
1. Spritz the inside of the cooker with cooking oil spray.
2. Whisk the flour, sweetener, coconut, salt, baking soda, and powdered egg whites in a large mixing container.
3. Add the coconut or almond milk, eggs, coconut extract, and melted coconut oil. Stir well and fold in the chips and berries.
4. Spread the prepared batter into the cooker and cook on the low setting for 3 hours. Turn the unit off and let it cool.
5. Top with whipped cream and serve.

Chapter 12: Smoothies & Fat Bombs

Smoothies

Almond Strawberry Smoothie

Yields Provided: 2 Servings
Nutritional Counts Per Serving:
- **Calories**: 304
- **Net Carbs**: 7 g
- **Total Fat Content**: 25 g
- **Protein**: 15 g

Ingredients Needed:
- Heavy cream (.5 cup)
- Unsweetened almond milk (16 oz.)
- Stevia (to taste)
- Frozen unsweetened strawberries (.25 cup)
- Whey vanilla isolate powder (2 tbsp.)

How to Prepare:
1. Toss or pour each of the fixings into a blender.
2. Puree until smooth.
3. Add a small amount of water to thin the smoothie as needed.

Avocado Almond Milk Smoothie

Yields Provided: 1 Serving

Nutritional Counts Per Serving:

- **Calories**: 587
- **Net Carbs**: 4 g
- **Total Fat Content**: 58 g
- **Protein**: 6 g

Ingredients Needed:

- Avocado (1)
- Unsweetened almond milk (3 oz.)
- Ice cubes (6)
- EZ-Sweetz sweetener/your preference (6 drops)
- Coconut cream (3 oz.)

How to Prepare:

1. Slice the avocado lengthwise before removing the seeds and the skin.
2. Toss the avocado with the rest of the fixings into the blender.
3. Add ice cubes and blend until smooth.

Avocado Mocha Smoothies

Yields Provided: 3 Servings
Nutritional Counts Per Serving:
- **Calories**: 176
- **Net Carbs**: 4 g
- **Total Fat Content**: 16 g
- **Protein**: 3 g

Ingredients Needed:
- Avocado (1)
- Cocoa powder - unsweetened (3 tbsp.)
- Plain almond milk (1.5 cups)
- Coconut milk – from the can (.5 cup)
- Vanilla extract (1 tsp.)
- Instant coffee crystals – regular or decaffeinated (2 tsp.)
- Erythritol blend/granulated stevia (3 tbsp.)

How to Prepare:
1. Use a sharp knife to slice the avocado in half and discard the pit.
2. Spoon out the fleshy center. Add it along with the rest of the ingredients into the blender.
3. Mix until smooth and serve.

Blackcurrant Smoothie

Yields Provided: 1 Serving
Nutritional Counts Per Serving:
- **Calories**: 228
- **Net Carbs**: 9 g
- **Total Fat Content**: 17 g
- **Protein**: 5 g

Ingredients Needed:
- Water (.5 cup)
- Frozen or fresh strawberries (.25 cup or 2-3 berries)
- Chia seeds - powdered or whole (2 tbsp.)
- Frozen or fresh blackcurrants (2.1 oz.)
- Heavy whipping cream/coconut milk (.25 cup)
- Sugar-free vanilla extract/1 vanilla bean (.5 tsp.)
- _Optional_: Stevia liquid (4-7 drops)

How to Prepare:
1. Toss all of the fixings into a blender.
2. Pulse until creamy. Wait for about five minutes for the flavors to mix.
3. Add ice either before or after mixing.

Blueberry Smoothie

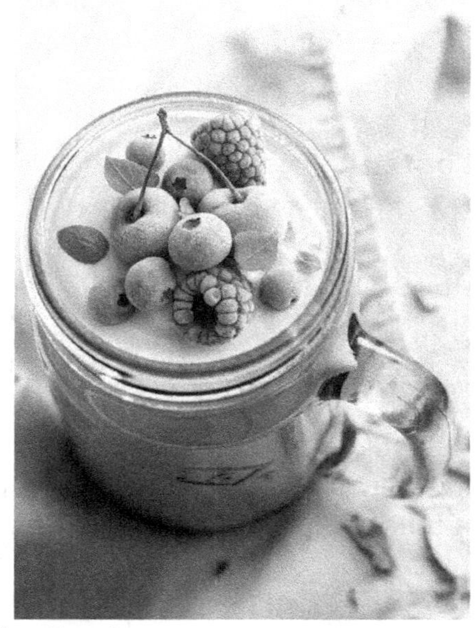

Yields Provided: 1 Serving
Nutritional Counts Per Serving:
- **Calories**: 215
- **Net Carbs**: 4 g
- **Total Fat Content**: 10 g
- **Protein**: 23 g

Ingredients Needed:
- Coconut milk or almond milk (1 cup)
- Blueberries (.25 cup)
- Vanilla extract (1 tsp.)
- MCT Oil or coconut oil (1 tsp.)
- *Optional:* Protein powder (30 g)

How to Prepare:
1. Put all the fixings into a blender. Blend until smooth.
2. Serve anytime for a delicious and healthy treat.

Blueberry & Kefir Smoothie

Yields Provided: 2 Servings
Nutritional Counts Per Serving:
- **Calories**: 476
- **Net Carbs**: 7 g
- **Total Fat Content**: 50 g
- **Protein**: 4 g

Ingredients Needed:
- Coconut milk kefir (1.5 cups)
- Fresh or frozen blueberries (.5 cup)
- MCT oil (2 tbsp.)
- Water (+) ice cubes (.5 cup)
- Sugar-free vanilla extract (1-2 tsp.) or pure vanilla powder (.5 tsp.)
- _Optional:_ Collagen powder (2 tbsp.)
- _Optional:_ Liquid stevia (3-5 drops)

How to Prepare:
1. Toss all of the ingredients into your blender
2. Pulse until the fixings are well mixed.
3. Serve in chilled glasses at breakfast to get your day started.

Cucumber & Spinach Smoothie

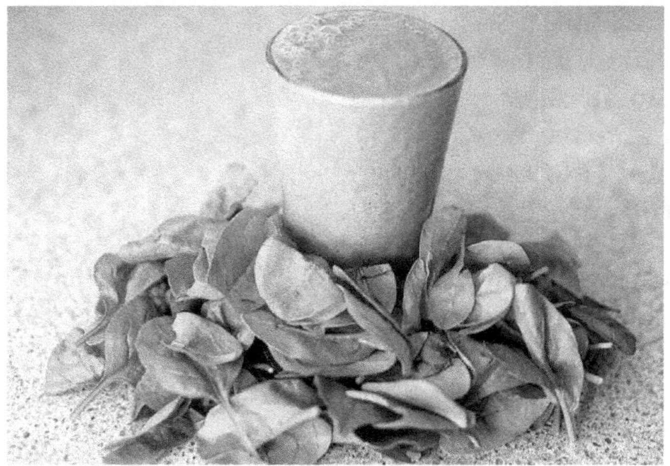

Yields Provided: 1 Serving

Nutritional Counts Per Serving:
- **Calories**: 330
- **Net Carbs**: 3 g
- **Total Fat Content**: 32 g
- **Protein**: 10 g

Ingredients Needed:
- Cucumber (2.5 oz.)
- Spinach (2 handfuls)
- Coconut milk from a carton (1 cup)
- Xanthan gum (.25 tsp.)
- MCT oil (1-2 tbsp.)
- Liquid stevia (12 drops)
- Large cubes of ice (7)

How to Prepare:
1. Peel and cube the cucumber. Add it and the remainder of the ingredients into a blender. Puree the mixture for 1-2 minutes.
2. Serve when ready.

Egg-Nog Smoothie

Yields Provided: 1 Serving
Nutritional Counts Per Serving:
- **Calories**: 320
- **Net Carbs**: 6 g
- **Total Fat Content**: 30 g
- **Protein**: 6 g

Ingredients Needed:
- Heavy whipping cream/coconut cream for dairy-free (.25 cup)
- Ground cloves (4 or .25 tsp.)
- Cinnamon (.5 tsp.)
- Large egg (1)
- Erythritol (1 tsp.)
- Sugar-free maple syrup (1 tsp.)

How to Prepare:
1. Place all ingredients into a blender.
2. Blend on high for 30 seconds to 1 minute or until frothy on top.
3. Serve.

Raspberry & Chocolate Cheesecake Smoothie

Yields Provided: 1 Serving
Nutritional Counts Per Serving:
- **Calories:** 512
- **Net Carbs:** 7 g
- **Total Fat Content:** 54 g
- **Protein:** 7 g

Ingredients Needed:
- Frozen or fresh raspberries (.33 cup)
- Heavy whipping cream/ Coconut milk (.25 cup)
- Full-fat cream cheese/creamed coconut milk (.25 cup)
- Unsweetened cacao powder (1 tbsp.)
- Extra-virgin coconut oil (1 tbsp.)
- Water (.5 cup)
- *Optional*: Liquid stevia extract (3-5 drops)

How to Prepare:
1. Toss all of the fixings in a blender.
2. Mix thoroughly until frothy.
3. Serve in a chilled glass.

St. Patrick's Day Smoothie

Yields Provided: 1 Serving
Nutritional Counts Per Serving:
- **Calories**: 493
- **Net Carbs**: 9 g
- **Total Fat Content**: 37 g
- **Protein**: 27 g

Ingredients Needed:
- Fresh baby spinach (.25 cup)
- Fresh mint/mint extract (as desired)
- Coconut milk or full-fat cream (.25 cup)
- Plain or vanilla whey protein/egg white protein powder (.25 cup)
- Medium avocado (3.5 oz. or .5 of 1)
- Vanilla bean (1) or (.5 - 1 tsp.) vanilla extract
- Unsalted pistachio nuts (2 tbsp.)
- Water (.5 cup)
- Liquid stevia extract (3-6 drops)
- Cubes of ice (5 or more)

How to Prepare:
1. Rinse the spinach and mint. Drain in a colander.
2. Cut the avocado in half. Mix all of the fixings in a blender.
3. Serve when frothy.
4. *Note:* Add some ice during or after you combine the smoothie.

Tropical Smoothie

Yields Provided: 2 Servings
Nutritional Counts Per Serving:
- **Calories:** 356
- **Net Carbs:** 4 g
- **Total Fat Content:** 33 g
- **Protein:** 4 g

Ingredients Needed:
- Golden flaxseed meal (2 tbsp.)
- Liquid stevia (20 drops)
- MCT oil (1 tbsp.)
- Blueberry extract (.25 tsp.)
- Banana extract (.25 tsp.)
- Mango extract (.5 tsp.)
- Unsweetened coconut milk (.75 cup)
- Sour cream (.25 cup)
- Large cubes of ice (7)
- *Also Needed:* NutriBullet or high-speed blender

How to Prepare:
1. Combine all of the fixings in your blender.
2. Wait a minute or two for the flax meal to soak some of the liquid.
3. Blend for one to two minutes until well mixed.
4. Serve and relax.

Fat Bombs

Salty

Cheesy Bacon Bombs

Yields Provided: 20 Servings
Nutritional Counts Per Serving:
- **Calories**: 89
- **Net Carbs**: 0.6 g
- **Total Fat Content**: 7 g
- **Protein**: 5 g

Ingredients Needed:
- Bacon (10 slices)
- Mozzarella cheese (8 oz.)
- Melted butter (4 tbsp.)
- Almond flour (4 tbsp.)
- Psyllium husk powder (3 tbsp.)
- Large egg (1)
- Sea salt (.25 tsp.)
- Black pepper (.25 tsp.)
- Onion powder (.125 tsp.)
- Garlic powder (.125 tsp.)
- Lard or oil for frying (1 cup)

How to Prepare:
1. Warm the oil/lard until it reaches 350° Fahrenheit in a pan or fryer.
2. Add about half the cheese into a microwavable dish and cook for 45 to 60 seconds until melted.
3. For the butter, microwave 15 to 20 seconds, and add to the cheese along with the egg.
4. Blend in the almond flour, psyllium husk, and spices. To make

prep easier, arrange the dough on a silicone mat and roll out into a rectangular shape.

5. Add the remainder of cheese and fold to form a rectangle. Slice into 20 squares.
6. Wrap each segment with 1/2 slice of bacon, and secure with a toothpick.
7. Cook each of the fat bombs (3-4 at a time) until crispy.
8. Remove to a paper-lined tray to drain. Serve.

Sweet

Almond Butter Fat Bombs

Yields Provided: 8 Servings
Nutritional Counts Per Serving:
- **Calories**: 145
- **Net Carbs**: 1.7 g
- **Total Fat Content**: 15 g
- **Protein**: 2 g

Ingredients Needed:
- Almond butter (9.5 tbsp.)
- Melted coconut oil (.75 cup)
- Liquid stevia (⅜ tsp. or 60 drops)
- Melted salted butter (9 tbsp.)
- Cocoa (3 tbsp.)

How to Prepare:
1. Combine all of the fixings until creamy smooth.
2. Pour into 24 mini muffin molds/silicone candy molds.
3. Freeze for at least 30 minutes. Pop them out and enjoy it for a delicious treat.

Almond & Pistachio Fat Bombs

Yields Provided: 36 Servings
Nutritional Counts Per Serving:
- **Calories**: 170
- **Net Carbs**: 3 g
- **Total Fat Content**: 17 g
- **Protein**: 2 g

Ingredients Needed:
- Full-fat coconut milk (.5 cup)
- Roasted almond butter (1 cup)
- Melted cacao butter (.5 cup)
- Firm coconut oil (1 cup)
- Creamy coconut butter (1 cup)
- Chai spice (2 tsp.)
- Ghee (.25 cup)
- Himalayan salt (.25 tsp.)
- Pure almond extract (.25 tsp.)
- Pure vanilla extract (1 tbsp.)
- Raw shelled pistachios (.25 tsp.)
- _Also Needed:_ 9-inch square baking pan

How to Prepare:
1. Chill the coconut milk overnight.
2. Grease the pan and line it with parchment paper.
3. Toss the butter into the microwave or saucepan to melt. Set aside for now.
4. Add everything except the pistachios, and cacao butter into a large bowl. Use the slow speed, and mix using a hand mixer until the mixture is airy and light.
5. Empty the melted cacao into the almond mix and continue mixing until it is well incorporated. Add it to the prepared pan and sprinkle using the chopped pistachios.
6. Refrigerate for at least four hours or overnight for best results.
7. Cut into 36 squares.

Avocado - PB - Chocolate Pudding Fat Bomb

Yields Provided: 1 Serving
Nutritional Counts Per Serving:
- **Calories**: 190
- **Net Carbs**: 2 g
- **Total Fat Content**: 13 g
- **Protein**: 2 g

Ingredients Needed:
- Ripe avocado (1)
- Stevia blend (1-2 tbsp.)
- Cocoa powder (1 tbsp.)
- MCT Oil Powder - ex Perfect Keto (1 scoop)
- Natural peanut butter (1 tbsp.)
- Unsweetened almond milk (.5 cup)
- Vanilla (.5 tsp.)

How to Prepare:
1. Peel and chop the avocado. Combine with the rest of the fixings.
2. Add small portions of almond milk until it's like you like it.
3. For the sweetener; begin with 1 tablespoon and add slowly to taste.
4. Serve.

Chocolate Fat Bombs

Yields Provided: 14 Servings
Nutritional Counts Per Serving:
- **Calories:** 119
- **Net Carbs:** 1 g
- **Total Fat Content:** 13 g
- **Protein:** 1.4 g

Ingredients Needed:
- Tahini paste (1-2 tbsp.)
- Unsweetened cocoa powder (1 oz.)
- Coconut oil (4.5 oz.)
- Your favorite granulated sweetener (1 tbsp.)
- Walnut halves - for decoration (1 oz.)

How to Prepare:
1. Melt the coconut oil along with the rest of the fixings in a saucepan (omit the walnuts).
2. Let the mixture cool slightly and pour into ice trays or candy molds.
3. Place in the fridge until mostly set. Add 1/2 of a walnut on each one before serving.

Cinnamon Coconut Bombs

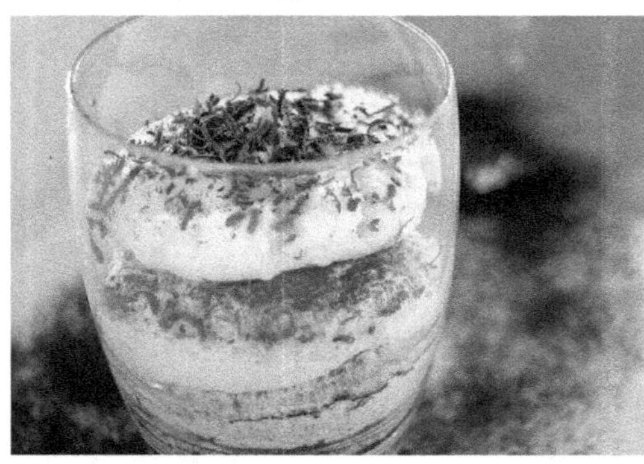

Yields Provided: 10 Servings

Nutritional Counts Per Serving:

- **Calories**: 341
- **Net Carbs**: 5 g
- **Total Fat Content**: 32 g
- **Protein**: 3 g

Ingredients Needed:

- Vanilla extract (1 tsp.)
- Canned coconut milk - full-fat (1 cup)
- Coconut butter (1 cup)
- Shredded coconut (1 cup)
- Cinnamon (.5 tsp.)
- Nutmeg (.5 tsp.)
- Stevia powder extract (1 tsp.) or Raw honey (2-3 tbsp. - count the extra carbs)

How to Prepare:

1. Prepare a double boiler and add all ingredients (omit the shredded coconut). Use medium heat until melted.
2. Let the mixture chill in the fridge for about 30 minutes.
3. Take the container out of the fridge and shape the mixture into ten balls. Roll them through the coconut pieces and refrigerate

for a minimum of one hour.

4.   Refrigerate until ready to eat.

Coconut & Blackberry Fat Bombs

Yields Provided: 16 Servings
Nutritional Counts Per Serving:
- **Calories**: 170
- **Net Carbs**: 3 g
- **Total Fat Content**: 19 g
- **Protein**: 1 g

Ingredients Needed:
- Coconut oil (1 cup)
- Coconut butter (1 cup)
- Fresh or frozen blackberries (.5 cup)
- Stevia drops (6 or to taste)
- Lemon juice (1 tbsp.)
- Vanilla extract (.5 tsp.)

How to Prepare:
1.   Add the coconut oil, coconut butter, and frozen berries in a cooking pot using the medium heat setting.
2.   Prepare the baking pan with a sheet of parchment baking paper.
3.   Blend and add the mixture (step 1) along with the rest of the components in the recipe.
4.   Spread it out on the prepared pan.
5.   Let them set in the fridge for about an hour.
6.   *Note:* If you use fresh berries, you won't need to cook them using the butter and coconut oil (step 1).

Coconut Orange Creamsicle Fat Bombs

Yields Provided: 10 Servings
Nutritional Counts Per Serving:
- **Calories**: 177
- **Net Carbs**: 0.95 g
- **Total Fat Content**: 19 g
- **Protein**: 1 g

Ingredients Needed:
- MiO Orange Vanilla (1 tsp.)
- Coconut oil (.5 cup)
- Cream cheese (4 oz.)
- Heavy whipping cream (.5 cup)
- Liquid stevia (10 drops)
- *Also Needed:* Immersion blender & Silicone tray

How to Prepare:
1. Blend all of the fixings together. If the mixture is too stiff, microwave it for a couple of seconds.
2. Spread the fixings into the tray and freeze for about two to three hours.
3. Once it's hardened, transfer to a container and store in the freezer until desired.
4. *Note*: Enjoy any of the flavors provided by the MiO water enhancer.

Coffee Fat Bombs

Yields Provided: 15 Servings
Nutritional Counts Per Serving:
- **Calories**: 45
- **Net Carbs**: 0 g
- **Total Fat Content**: 4 g
- **Protein**: 0 g

Ingredients Needed:
- Unchilled cream cheese (4.4 oz.)
- Powdered xylitol (2 tbsp.)
- Instant coffee (1 tbsp.)
- Unsweetened cocoa powder (1 tbsp.)
- Unchilled butter (1 tbsp.)
- Coconut oil (1 tbsp.)

How to Prepare:
1. With a blender/food processor to blitz the xylitol and coffee into a fine powder. Mix in the hot water to form a pasty mixture.
2. Blend in the cream cheese, cocoa powder, butter, and coconut oil.
3. Add to ice cube trays and freeze a minimum of one to two hours.
4. Use a zipper-type baggie to keep them fresh in the freezer.

Strawberry Cheesecake Fat Bombs

Yields Provided: 12 Servings
Nutritional Counts Per Serving:
- **Calories:** 67
- **Net Carbs:** 0.85 g
- **Total Fat Content:** 7 g
- **Protein:** 1 g

Ingredients Needed:
- Softened - Unchilled cream cheese - _don't microwave_ (.75 cup)
- Coconut oil or softened butter (.25 cup)
- Fresh/frozen strawberries (.5 cup)
- Liquid stevia (10-15 drops) or Powdered erythritol (2 tbsp.)
- Vanilla extract (1 tbsp.)

How to Prepare:
1. Mix the butter or coconut oil with the cream cheese in a mixing container.
2. Prepare the berries and remove the stems. Add them to a dish and mash until smooth. Stir in the stevia and vanilla. (Mix well using a food processor or hand whisk.)
3. Scoop out the mixture and add into candy molds or muffin silicone molds.
4. Let the bombs rest in the freezer until set; usually about two hours.
5. Just pop them out and serve.

Tiramisu Fat Bombs

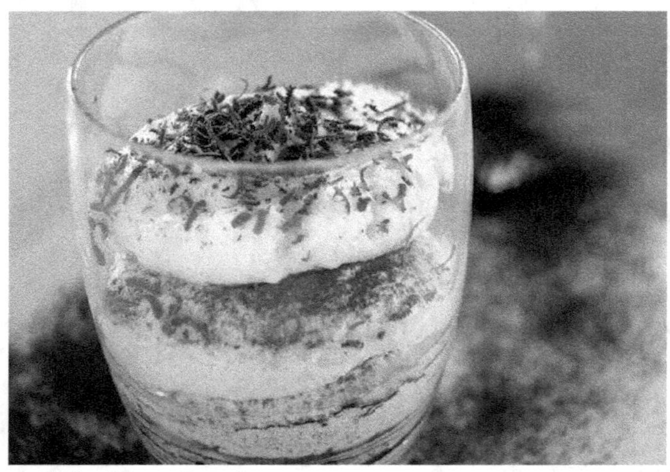

Yields Provided: 24 Servings
Nutritional Counts Per Serving:
- **Calories**: 75
- **Net Carbs**: 0.8 g
- **Total Fat Content**: 7 g
- **Protein**: 1.2 g

Ingredients Needed:
- Coconut flour (.25 cup + 2 tbsp.)
- Classic monk fruit sweetener - divided (.25 cup)
- Cinnamon (.125 or to your liking)
- Hot water (.5 cup)
- Melted butter (.25 cup)
- Espresso powder (2 tsp.)
- Unchilled cream cheese (4 oz.)
- Unchilled butter (.25 cup)
- Unchilled No-Sugar-Added SunButter (.25 cup)
- Pinot noir (1 tbsp.)
- Pure vanilla extract (1 tsp.)
- Cocoa powder (.75 cup)

How to Prepare:

1. In a small saucepan, using the medium temperature setting, toast the coconut flour until golden and fragrant, about five minutes, stirring frequently.
2. Whisk the toasted flour, 1 tbsp. sweetener, and cinnamon together.
3. Pour in hot water, melted butter, and espresso. Mix with a fork until well-incorporated. Spoon the mixture into silicone mold cavities and, using your fingers, press into an even layer. Transfer the mold into the freezer to chill.
4. Meanwhile, add the cream cheese, butter, SunButter, remaining 3 tbsp. sweetener, pinot noir, and vanilla extract. Mix the fixings until thoroughly combined using an electric mixer. Cover the mixing container with a lid or plastic wrap. Chill for 15 minutes.
5. After the cream cheese mixture has chilled, remove the mold from the freezer, and spoon the cream cheese mixture into the molds - atop the crust mixture. Sprinkle cocoa powder on top.
6. Return the mold to the freezer until the fat bombs are solid. They can be easily popped out in about two hours.

Ice Cream

Blueberry Coconut & Lime Ice Cream

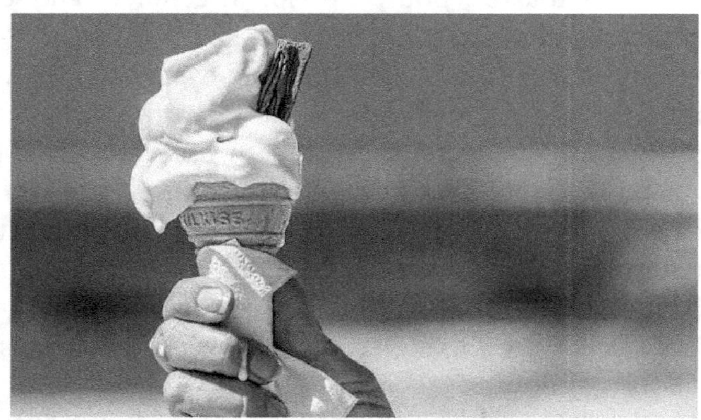

Yields Provided: 8 Servings
Nutritional Counts Per Serving:
- **Calories**: 185
- **Net Carbs**: 3.5 g
- **Total Fat Content**: 14 g
- **Protein**: 1 g

Ingredients Needed:
- Lime juice (1 lime)
- White sweetener - erythritol or inulin (.66 cup)
- Blueberries (1 cup)
- Coconut cream (13.5 oz. can)
- Unsweetened almond milk or coconut milk (.33 cup)
- *Optional:* Xanthan gum (.5 tsp.)

How to Prepare:
1. Squeeze the juice and zest from the lime into a saucepan.
2. Whisk the cream layer from the canned coconut cream until stiff peaks form.

3. Pour the liquid part of the coconut cream, sweetener, blueberries, and low carb milk into the pan with the lime prep.
4. Heat to boiling and gently simmer for approximately four minutes.
5. Transfer to the countertop and whisk in the xanthan gum. Cool slightly and fold in the whipped coconut cream.
6. Chill in the fridge until cool.
7. Process in an ice cream maker and serve.

Cheesecake Popsicles

Yields Provided: 12 Servings
Nutritional Counts Per Serving:
- **Calories**: 122
- **Net Carbs**: 3 g
- **Total Fat Content**: 12 g
- **Protein**: 2 g

Ingredients Needed:
- Unchilled cream cheese (8 oz.)
- Cream (1 cup)
- Chopped strawberries (2 cups)
- Powdered swerve (.33 cup)
- Stevia extract (.25 tsp.)
- Lemon juice (1 tbsp.)
- *Also Needed*:
- 12 wooden sticks
- Popsicle mold

How to Prepare:
1. Take the cream cheese out of the fridge to soften for 30 minutes - minimum. Add to a food processor and pulse until smooth.
2. Pour in the cream, stevia, swerve, and juice. Mix well.
3. Add the berries (.5 of 1 cup at a time).
4. Pour each one into a popsicle mold with a wooden stick.
5. Freeze for at least four hours.

Chocolate Ice Cream

Yields Provided: 2 Servings
Nutritional Counts Per Serving:
- **Calories**: 177
- **Net Carbs**: 3 g
- **Total Fat Content**: 14 g
- **Protein**: 3 g

Ingredients Needed:
- Eggs (4)
- Egg yolks - in addition to the whole eggs (4 or 5)
- Apple cider vinegar/Lemon juice (1 tsp.)
- Melted butter/ghee (7 tbsp.)
- Melted cacao butter (3.5 tbsp.)
- XCT oil (6 tbsp. + 1 scant tsp.)
- Melted coconut oil (3 tbsp. + 2 tsp.)
- Granulated sweetener of choice (3.5 tbsp./as desired)
- Filtered water or ice (just under .25 cup)
- Cocoa powder (.25 or .33 cup)
- Vanilla powder (2 tsp.)
- _Optional:_ Cinnamon (1-2 tsp.)
- _Also Needed:_ High-powered blender & Ice cream maker

How to Prepare:
1. Toss all of the fixings into the blender.
2. Mix for one to two minutes or until combined.
3. Taste test and adjust the sweetness to your preference.
4. Empty the mixture into the ice cream maker.
5. Churn for approximately 15 to 20 minutes before serving.

Creamy Key Lime Popsicles

Yields Provided: 6 Servings
Nutritional Counts Per Serving:
- **Calories**: 264
- **Net Carbs**: 5 g
- **Total Fat Content**: 26 g
- **Protein**: 3 g

Ingredients Needed:
- Large ripe avocados (2)
- Organic zest (1 lime)
- Juice (2 limes)
- Coconut milk (15 oz.)
- Swerve or powdered erythritol (.5 cup/2.8 oz.)
- Liquid stevia (15-20 drops)
- *Also Needed:* Popsicle sticks and molds

How to Prepare:
1. Use a sharp knife to slice the avocados into halves and remove the seeds. Spoon the pulp into a mixing container.
2. Prepare the zest of lime and mix in with the juice, coconut milk, powdered erythritol, and stevia.
3. Mix until smooth using a hand mixer. Spoon out the mixture and add to the popsicle molds.
4. Insert a stick into each of one and freeze for a minimum of three to four hours or until solid.

Peanut Butter Ice Cream

Yields Provided: 8 Servings
Nutritional Counts Per Serving:
- **Calories**: 378
- **Net Carbs**: 4 g
- **Total Fat Content**: 26 g
- **Protein**: 10 g

Ingredients Needed:
- Swerve (.5 cup)
- Stevia extract powder (.25 tsp.)
- *Optional:* Monk fruit powder (.25 tsp.)
- *Optional:* Natural whey protein (.25 cup)
- Salt (.125 tsp.)
- Peanut butter - natural organic/half creamy - half chunky (1 cup)
- Unsweetened almond milk (1 cup)
- Heavy cream (1.33 cups)
- Xanthan gum (.25 tsp.)
- Vanilla extract (2 tsp.)

How to Prepare:
1. Mix the stevia, peanut butter, salt, and monk fruit, and whey protein.
2. Whisk or blend the xanthan gum and milk.
3. Stir in vanilla and heavy cream.
4. Add the fixings to an ice cream maker and process to your liking.

<u>Raspberry Ice Cream</u>

Yields Provided: 5 Servings
Nutritional Counts Per Serving:
- **Calories:** 183
- **Net Carbs:** 3 g
- **Total Fat Content:** 16 g
- **Protein:** 1 g

Ingredients Needed:
- Heavy cream (or coconut cream (1 cup)
- Frozen raspberries (2 cups)
- Powdered erythritol or any sweetener (.33 cup or to your liking)

How to Prepare:
1. Pour the cream into a blender. Blend until stiff peaks form (you can also use a hand mixer if your blender isn't powerful enough to whip the cream).
2. Toss the frozen raspberries and sweetener into the blender. Puree until incorporated. Adjust the sweetener to taste if needed, and if added, puree again.
3. This ice cream is a soft-serve consistency. For firmer ice cream; run the mixture through an ice cream maker, or place in the freezer to firm up.
4. (For the freezer, stir every 30-60 minutes for the first couple hours to break up any ice crystals.)

Strawberry Coconut Ice Cream

Yields Provided: 6 Large Servings
Nutritional Counts Per Serving:
- **Calories**: 327
- **Net Carbs**: 6.9 g
- **Total Fat Content**: 38.2 g
- **Protein**: 3.9 g

Ingredients Needed:
- Full-fat coconut milk, using both water and coconut cream (4 cups)
- Erythritol (.5 cup)
- Chopped strawberries (8 oz. - divided)

How to Prepare:
1. Add the coconut milk, erythritol and half of the strawberries to a food processor/blender. If you are adding MCT oil or vodka, add it now.
2. Blend using the high setting until smooth.
3. Fold in the rest of the strawberries.
4. Prepare a loaf pan or another freezer-safe container of choice with parchment baking paper. Pour the ice cream into the pan.
5. Cover tightly with aluminum foil and freeze for 2 to 3 hours. Serve.
6. Leftover ice cream may need a few minutes on the counter to re-soften after freezing.

Chapter 13: Special Menu Plan

You can enjoy each of the recipes listed in your new meal plan since each one has the net carbs per serving posted. You will see how flexible the plan is when you look at how easy it is to use just the recipes in this cookbook for 21 full days including 3 meals, snacks, or dessert.

You can also enjoy other delicious tasty desserts and snacks at any time of the day or night. According to a favorite source: you should maintain the carb levels between 20 (optimal effect) to 50 net carbs daily.

Keep in mind, these are suggestions and can be changed according to your schedule. All you need to do is count the carbs as provided with each of the selections throughout your new cookbook. Please enjoy!

Day 1:
Breakfast: Bagels with Cheese: 8 g
Lunch: Tuna Salad & Chives: 1 g
Dinner: Nacho Chicken Casserole: 4.3 g
Snack or Dessert: Raspberry Ice Cream: 3 g
Day 2:
Breakfast: Sausage Hot Pockets: 6.6 g
Lunch: Egg Drop Soup: 3 g
Dinner: Beetroot-Cured Salmon with Dill Oil: 4 g
Snack or Dessert: Cranberry Bliss Cookies: 2 g
Day 3:
Breakfast: Blueberry Ricotta Pancakes: 6 g
Lunch: Cauliflower & Rice Salad: 1 g
Dinner: Chicken Asparagus Dinner: 4 g
Snack or Dessert: Chocolate Hazelnut Tarts: 3 g
Day 4:
Breakfast: Ham Cheese Soufflé: 5 g

Lunch: Chicken-Pecan Salad & Cucumber Bites: 3 g
Dinner: Shrimp Alfredo: 6.5 g
Snack or Dessert: Chocolate Ice Cream: 3 g
Day 5:
Breakfast: Blueberry Hemp Seed Breakfast Oatmeal: 5 g
Lunch: Vegetarian Club Salad: 5 g
Dinner: BBQ Flank Steak: 1 g & Cauliflower Mac & Cheese: 7 g
Snack or Dessert: Coconut Cream Brownies: 2
Day 6:
Breakfast: Brunch Tomato Pesto Mug Cake: 4 g
Lunch: Keto Salad Niçoise: 8 g
Dinner: Pesto & Mozzarella Chicken Casserole: 3 g
Snack or Dessert: Cinnamon Coconut Bombs: 5 g
Day 7:
Breakfast: Eggs & Mackerel Brunch Plate: 4 g
Lunch: Salad Sandwiches: 3 g
Dinner: Slow-Cooked Chuck Steak: 3 g & Asparagus & Garlic: 2 g
Snack or Dessert: Cheesecake Popsicles: 3 g
Day 8:
Breakfast: Cocoa Waffles: 3.4 g
Lunch: King-Sized Keto Salad: 9 g
Dinner: Fettuccine Chicken Alfredo: 1 g
Snack or Dessert: Apple & Carrot Spice Walnut Cake: 4 g
Day 9:
Breakfast: Avocado & Bacon Omelet: 3.3 g
Lunch: Caprese Salad: 5 g
Dinner: Jamaican Jerk Pork Roast: 0 g & Broccoli & Cheese Casserole: 2 g
Snack or Dessert: Banana Split Cheesecake: 7 g
Day 10:
Breakfast: Bacon Hash: 9 g
Lunch: Grilled Chicken Salad: 0.8 g
Dinner: Ground Beef Veggie Skillet: 6 g
Snack or Dessert: Peanut Butter Ice Cream: 4 g
Day 11:
Breakfast: Almond - Coconut Egg Wraps: 3 g

Lunch: Greek Salad: 8 g

Dinner: Slow-Cooked Teriyaki: 4 g

Snack or Dessert: Chocolate Lava Cake: 3 g

Day 12:

Breakfast: Pumpkin Spice Waffles: 5 g

Lunch: Jar Salad with Tempeh - Vegan: 4 g

Dinner: Pimiento Cheese Meatballs: 1 g & Garlic Parmesan Fried Eggplant: 6 g

Snack or Dessert: Orange Cream Cheese Cookies & Nuts: 2 g

Day 13:

Breakfast: Cream Cheese Eggs: 3 g

Lunch: Chicken Cauliflower Rice Soup: 7 g

Dinner: Slow-Cooked London Broil: 2.5 g & Asparagus & Garlic: 2 g

Snack or Dessert: Strawberry Cheesecake Fat Bombs: 0.85

Day 14:

Breakfast: Brunch BLT Wrap: 2 g

Lunch: Pan-Fried Peach Scallops Salad: 7 g

Dinner: Creamy Chicken & Greens: 3 g

Snack or Dessert: Blueberry Coconut & Lime Ice Cream: 3.5 g

Day 15:

Breakfast: Green Buttered Eggs: 2.5 g

Lunch: No-Beans Beef Chili: 8 g

Dinner: Baked Tilapia with Cherry Tomatoes: 4 g

Snack or Dessert: Creamy Key Lime Popsicles: 5 g

Day 16:

Breakfast: Belgian Style Waffles: 3 g

Lunch: Shrimp Avocado Salad with Tomatoes & Feta: 6.5 g

Dinner: Jamaican Jerk Pork Roast: 0 g & Bacon-Wrapped Mushrooms: 1.6 g

Snack or Dessert: Egg-Nog Smoothie: 6 g

Day 17:

Breakfast: Cheesy Italian Omelet: 3 g

Lunch: Crockpot Chicken Chowder: 7.5 g

Dinner: Lamb Chops with Herb Butter: 0.3 g (2 recipes)

Snack or Dessert: Strawberry Coconut Ice Cream: 6.9 g

Day 18:

Breakfast: Creamy Basil Baked Sausage: 4 g

Lunch: Spring Soup with Poached Egg: 4 g

Dinner: Avocado & Salmon Omelet Wrap: 6 g & Creamy Asparagus Soup: 3 g

Snack or Dessert: Blueberry Smoothie: 4 g

Day 19:

Breakfast: Lemon Waffles: 1.8 g

Lunch: Avocado - Corn Salad: 11 g

Dinner: Rotisserie Chicken & Cabbage Shreds: 6 g

Snack or Dessert: Coconut Orange Creamsicle Fat Bombs: 0.95 g

Day 20:

Breakfast: Blueberry Hemp Seed Breakfast Oatmeal: 5 g

Lunch: Cobb Salad: 3 g

Dinner: Pulled Pork Hash: 8 g & Broccoli & Cheese Casserole: 2 g

Snack or Dessert: Cheesecake Pudding: 5 g

Day 21:

Breakfast: Brunch Tomato Pesto Mug Cake: 4 g

Lunch: Greens Soup: 6 g

Dinner: Beef Cabbage Soup: 4 g & Cheeseburger Calzone: 3 g

Snack or Dessert: Blueberry Bar: 7 g

You should have the basics of how to plan your meals using your new cookbook and guidelines. As you see, each of the recipes falls into the category of between 20 and 50 net carbs as used with the ketogenic diet plan. You can add to the meal plan according to the number of carbs you choose for your 'personal' plan.

Conclusion

I hope you have already enjoyed several of the meals provided in *Keto Diet Cookbook 2020* I hope it was also informative and provided you with all of the tools you need to achieve your goals - whatever they may be.

You will need to understand how to maintain your ketosis status while you are enjoying your delicious recipes. There are several methods used to monitor your ketone activity and stay in line with your dieting goals. The levels of beta-hydroxybutyrate, acetone, and acetoacetate can be measured in your urine, breath, and blood.

Test your urine for acetoacetate. The strip is dipped into the urine which will change the color of the strip. The various shades of purple and pink indicate the levels of ketones. The darker the color on the testing strip; the higher the level of ketones. The major benefit is they are inexpensive. The most effective time to test is early in the morning after a ketogenic diet dinner the evening before testing.

Measure the ketones with a blood ketone meter. All it takes is a small drop of blood on a testing strip inserted into the meter. This process has been researched as an excellent indicator of your current ketosis levels. Unfortunately, the testing strips are expensive.

Lastly, use a Ketonix meter to measure your breath. You breathe into the meter. The results will be provided by a special coded color that will flash to show your levels of ketosis at that time.

At first, you may not notice the weight loss. There could be days or weeks where you don't see the changes, but slow is the best method. You are altering your lifestyle and breaking old habits. You need to remain patient because there aren't any quick fixes to weight loss. As with any new challenge, the initial phase of a long-term trial is difficult.

You have to realize the adoption time of the ketogenic diet plan can take anywhere from two to four weeks or more. For some, it can take as much as six to eight weeks. It takes time because you cannot instantly switch over to using fat as a fuel source. It takes time for your body to adjust to the changes. You may be experiencing low energy, withdrawal-type symptoms, fatigue or headaches, but they will pass.

Make use of your slow cooker or crockpot, food processor, and an immersion blender to prepare delicious meals using your ketogenic meal plan. Some recipes might not be 100 % keto-friendly. You can also adjust the ingredients to your own discretion. Remember this Formula: Total Carbs minus (-) Fiber = Net Carbs. This is the logic used for each of the recipes included in this cookbook and guidelines.

Finally, if you found this book useful in any way, a review on Amazon is always appreciated!

Index for The Recipes

- BBQ Chicken Zucchini Boats
- Cashew Chicken Curry
- Chicken Asparagus Dinner
- Chicken Nuggets
- Creamy Chicken & Greens
- Curry Chicken Lettuce Wraps
- Fettuccine Chicken Alfredo
- Nacho Chicken Casserole
- Pesto & Mozzarella Chicken Casserole
- Rotisserie Chicken & Cabbage Shreds
- Slow-Cooked Teriyaki

Chapter 5: Dinner: Seafood Selections

- Avocado & Salmon Omelet Wrap
- Baked Tilapia with Cherry Tomatoes
- Beetroot-Cured Salmon with Dill Oil
- Chipotle Fish Tacos
- Cod - Skillet Fried
- Fish Cakes
- Garlic & Lemon Shrimp Pasta
- Sesame Ginger Salmon
- Shrimp Alfredo
- Tangy Shrimp

Chapter 6: Dinner: Beef Options

- Bacon Cheeseburger
- BBQ Flank Steak
- Cheeseburger Calzone
- Feta-Stuffed Burgers
- Ground Beef Veggie Skillet
- Pimiento Cheese Meatballs

- Slow-Cooked - Chuck Steak
- Slow-Cooked London Broil
- Steak Pinwheels

Chapter 7: Dinner: Pork - Lamb & Other Favorites

- Jamaican Jerk Pork Roast
- Keto Pork Kabobs
- Luau Pork with Cauli Rice
- Pulled Pork Hash
- Stuffed Pork Chops

Lamb Options

- Lamb Chops with Herb Butter (2 recipes)
- Lamb Curry
- Roasted Leg of Lamb

Other Options

- Garlic Parmesan Sausage Skillet

Chapter 8: Side Dishes

- Asparagus & Garlic
- Broccoli & Cheese Casserole
- Cauliflower Mac & Cheese
- Garlic Parmesan Fried Eggplant

Chapter 9: Appetizers

- Air Fried - Bacon-Wrapped Chicken

- Bacon-Wrapped Mozzarella Sticks
- Cheese-Stuffed Bacon-Wrapped Hot Dogs
- Mortadella & Brie Plate
- Pita Pizza
- Salmon & Cream Cheese Bites

Chapter 10: Snack Options

Sweet Choices

- Choco Mug Brownie
- Chocolate Biscotti
- Chocolate Zucchini Cookies
- Cinnamon Coconut Chips
- Orange Cream Cheese Cookies & Nuts
- Peanut Butter & Coconut Balls
- Pistachio Cookies

Salty Choices
- Bacon Cheddar Cheese Crisps
- Bacon Knots
  Bacon-Wrapped Mushrooms
  Beef Pizza
- Cheese Chips
- Cheese Puffs
- Cheese Wraps
- Fried Queso Fresco
- Nut-Free Keto Crackers
- Olive Cheese Balls
- Roasted Almonds
- Roasted Pumpkin Seeds
- Slow-Roasted Cashews

Chapter 11: Desserts

- Apple & Carrot Spice Walnut Cake

- Banana Split Cheesecake
- Blueberry Bar
- Caramel Cake
- Cheesecake Pudding
- Chocolate Hazelnut Tarts
- Chocolate Lava Cake
- Coconut Cream Brownies
- Cranberry Bliss Cookies
  Raspberry Coconut Cake – Slow-Cooked

Chapter 12: Smoothies - Fat Bombs & Ice Cream

Smoothies

- Almond Strawberry Smoothie
- Avocado Almond Milk Smoothie
- Avocado Mocha Smoothies
- Blackcurrant Smoothie
- Blueberry Smoothie
- Blueberry & Kefir Smoothie
- Cucumber & Spinach Smoothie
- Egg-Nog Smoothie
- Raspberry & Chocolate Cheesecake Smoothie
- St. Patrick's Day Smoothie
- Tropical Smoothie

Fat Bombs

Salty

- Cheesy Bacon Bombs

Sweet

- Almond Butter Fat Bombs

- Almond & Pistachio Fat Bombs
- Avocado - PB - Chocolate Pudding Fat Bomb
- Chocolate Fat Bombs
- Cinnamon Coconut Bombs
- Coconut & Blackberry Fat Bombs
- Coconut Orange Creamsicle Fat Bombs
- Coffee Fat Bombs
- Strawberry Cheesecake Fat Bombs
- Tiramisu Fat Bombs

Ice Cream

- Blueberry Coconut & Lime Ice Cream
- Cheesecake Popsicles
- Chocolate Ice Cream
- Creamy Key Lime Popsicles
- Peanut Butter Ice Cream
- Raspberry Ice Cream
- Strawberry Coconut Ice Cream